"Sally Hughes Smith's moving account of one family's profound transition as they face their mother's dementia is surprisingly hopeful. Filled with honest emotions and personal details, *The Circle* is an inside look at a journey most of us dread. Ms. Smith shows us how to do it right!"

- *Marjory Wentworth, Poet Laureate of South Carolina*

"I had the pleasure of reading Sally Smith's *The Circle*. I've read a number of narratives describing the experiences of children and spouses who have cared for someone with Alzheimer's disease and I found Sally Smith's story to be unique in several ways. Clearly, this is written from the perspective of a child who had a close relationship with her mother and siblings, but most important, it presents both the challenges and experiences in an appropriately positive way. It doesn't downplay the difficulties nor does it present issues in a saccharin manner. Rather, it illustrates that caregiving and decision making for a person with progressive dementia has both light and dark moments, challenges and benefits, tears and laughter."

- *Peter V. Rabins, M.D., Professor of Psychiatry, Johns Hopkins University*

"Poignant and direct, beautiful and honest, *The Circle* brims with universal themes and generosity of spirit."

- *Barbara G.S. Hagerty, author of Purse Universe and Handbags*

THE CIRCLE

A Walk with Dementia

Sally Hughes Smith

Heartfelt thanks to the many who came
together to make this happen,
too many to name — you know who you are.
Special thanks for Debbie Bordeau's orchestration and
Virginia Beach's editing in the home stretch.

Library of Congress Control Number:
2006902658

ISBN 0-9779235-0-9

$20.00
All proceeds benefit medical research.
Available at special quantity discount
for purchase; contact:

Website address: www.musc.edu/aging

or Call (843) 792-0712

Printed in the United States of America
Medical University of South Carolina

First Edition

Book design by
Teresa Hilton
Printing Services, Medical University of South Carolina

Dear Reader,

The Center on Aging is excited to have an opportunity to take a unique narrative and produce something that will not only be a useful tool for families of dementia patients, but support research towards a cure as well. Proceeds from the sale of this book will support research into Parkinson's and Alzheimer's diseases, dementia, vision and hearing loss, and other age-related problems.

The Circle is a moving and personal story told with heart. I picked it up to read a quick page or two, dropped everything and couldn't put it down. Others have felt the same. I would like to share a sampling of quotes about it from different people.

"I used it like a map and I stayed connected. / . . . a balm for fractured families; / What there is on this subject is dismal —what a joy to read something positive. / There is strength in the honesty—required reading for our age group! / This is a subject that touches us all. / I'm a grown man and I have to admit I teared up."

There is a need for such a book. Soon, ten thousand people will turn sixty-five *every day* in the United States. However, only five titles were found for sale in the section on aging, dementia, and Alzheimer's disease on a recent trip to one of our national bookstore chains.

The Center on Aging at the Medical University of South Carolina is searching for meaningful new therapies for those ailments most commonly suffered by patients over sixty. Through publication of *The Circle*, we hope to aid more families, increase the awareness of our work on age-related problems, and support the research pivotal to creating a better quality of life for those facing the serious challenges of aging in our society.

Lotta Granholm-Bentley, D.D.S., Ph.D.
Director, Center on Aging
Medical University of South Carolina

FOREWORD

This is a tale about those—all of us really—left behind when someone we love leaves us to our lives—in their very midst—as a result either of cognitive decline or dementia. Any family similarly affected will grapple with many of the same issues as those faced by the Hughes family, and some will have to deal with decidedly more difficult decisions.

Many of the post World War II babies are confronting these challenges now as their parents move from being fully capable, independent persons to ones needing some level of assistance daily.

The Circle, a diary of days with events both mundane and profound leading up to a new existence for Mother at The Gardens, is an intimate and personal telling by Sally of her own journey and of the terms by which she coped with a mother's cognitive decline and the symptoms of dementia. Her words are intended to place us there in her childhood home as this particular tapestry frays and is repaired as best can be. It is a "you're not in this alone" story as we the readers in our own spaces deal with the imminent loss of someone dear to us or more precisely the loss of "the who and what they once were." The home as a metaphor for a life's time is well used here as this tightly knit family returns to and takes leave of the home their parents built. Parents generally, and here specifically Dr. Jimmy and Jane Hughes, impart much—often wordlessly—to us as we their offspring grow into adulthood. Those values, too, are on display here. *The Circle* is a good read; the emotional and physical ups and downs of the family will resonate with many outside their tiny circle.

The shell of who they once were is what we see when we visit our own mothers and fathers in their "Gardens," but what will be remembered and revered about them for the rest of our own time are the vignettes like Sally's. We've inherited and hold more in our hearts and minds than an arm load of hats or organdy gowns salvaged from the attic—we are who we are today because of who and what they, our parents, were then. These are stories that many families, regrettably, are writing in their own words today and will write for many tomorrows to come.

Stephan Snyder, Ph.D., National Institute on Aging, Program Director

DEDICATION

Our family is a circle of
          love and strength.
With every birth and every
          union, the circle grows.
Every joy shared adds more
          love.
Every crisis faced together
          makes the circle stronger.
                    -Anonymous

This journal is dedicated to my brother, Allen,
and sisters, Jane and Anne, with love and
gratitude for a lifetime of being there, for their
big hearts, integrity, loyalty, and all of the sheer
fun of our times together growing up and
always.

THE CIRCLE

A Walk with Dementia

_____

Sally Hughes Smith

_____

INTRODUCTION

Sometimes things take on a life of their own. This personal journal and its aftermath are certainly proof of that.

Like so many of our baby boom generation, my siblings and I have had to deal with the elusive realities and poignant choices in moving a beloved parent from a once vibrant "heart home" into an assisted living facility. In doing so, I serendipitously wrote this journal, putting down my thoughts as they came, never intending to see it in print. As I shared it with my family and a few close friends, they, in turn, began to share it with others. It began to spread. Soon I was getting the most amazing and totally unsolicited responses. What became apparent was that *The Circle* touched people who are also trying to deal positively with aging loved ones and don't really know that much about the terrain. "This must be published!" was the overriding message.

Having written the journal in a deeply personal way, the idea of sharing it beyond my circle of acquaintances was a foreign thought. I felt as though I would be baring my soul to the world. However, as people continued to express how it had helped them, I began to see that I had an opportunity to perhaps make a difference to people on a tough journey, people I didn't even know. What are we living for if we cannot be brave enough to do that? I have become brave. Part of what made me that way is that, though the story has many layers, it is ultimately about love. In our fractured world, any touch of that is welcome. Thus, you see *The Circle* before you.

I find that there is very little guidance available in this field, despite much interest in it. My journal is a true story of how one family did its best with their mother, with transition, and with the passage through this final stage of their own growing up. My uncle, writer Andrew Lytle, told me many times that once a creative work is "loosed on the world, it is too late for explanations." Yet, I take a moment to ask that you forgive the broad brushstrokes of the writing technique natural to a journal, moving beyond that to the feelings that ring true. I wrote it as my feelings flowed and have left it in this fresh, raw form, feeling it is strongest this way. I share this personal diary with you in the simple hope that it will be of use to you on your own journey.

We are all connected.

Sally Hughes Smith

WHO'S WHO IN 2001

Jane and Dr. Jimmy Hughes
(Jimmy has died in 2000 at age 89).
Their four children and their families as
of the date of Mother's move:

Dr. Allen & Marily	Jane & Bill	Sally & Dr. C.D.	Anne & Robert
Allen Jr. & Laurie	Elizabeth	Donovan & Ellen	Bob
Mary Catherine	Anne & David	*Cecilia*	Jim
Caroline		Whitney & Brooks	Janie
Allen III		Taylor	
Catherine & Dick		Langdon	
Will			

1
FIRST TRIP BACK HOME

This particular journey is part of a circle. It is the time when I am beginning to be one of the unravelers of a beautiful but strong tapestry that was woven over my lifetime. I guess that is not really right. I'm here to unravel a part of that tapestry, the physical part, my childhood home, and at the same time to patch a part of it—a very important part of it—my mother's last hope at a cheery, good few years as she sweetly walks into senility. That last chance means moving outside these big beautiful walls into an action filled, people filled, open armed homeplace. It means enjoying my mother these last few days here as she is more the child and I the parent. The circle. She wandered into her old master bedroom where sister Jane and I were asleep about four o'clock this predawn and Jane got her to come in between us and settle down to sleep. I was lying there in the dark thinking of the ironies. There we were in the very bed where we were both conceived with our mother between us. The one from whose body we had sprung. She was fidgeting with the covers, carefully smoothing the sheets, tucking us in, fussing over us quietly. We'll never be like this again. This particular circle is coming to completion and we will be part of our own family circles and perhaps someday lie between our own offspring on the eve of a great change.

I grew up in this place, with these things, with these people (except for Daddy who is gone, but who doesn't seem gone—especially when I talk out loud to him). This house has good bones. It was built when Mother and Daddy were on the threshold of making their lives something and were thinking big. Full of life. "Headlong Hall," Daddy called it. It has always had good vibes. No ugly secrets. No tragedies—just full, rich, human life. The next owners will feel it, I bet. I can say things like that now as I begin to accept letting it go, not just with my lips and mind, but honestly and realistically with all of me. I was thinking that tonight when I was taking a long soaky bath in Mother and Daddy's blue bathroom. I looked at the baby blue tiles, still pristine, grout and all, after fifty something years. I remembered my Mother bathing there on a hot summer afternoon before we had air conditioning and when I was little. I remember her head of short dark curly hair and how she unruffledly covered herself in the water, not reprimanding, when I burst in the door without knocking following some backyard excitement I ran to tell her about.

That bathroom, too, was the scene of lots of early morning visits with my charismatic father. He always played the news on the radio when he shaved. He had maps taped to the mirror of foreign countries where global events were unfolding. (Later it was vocabulary words—French, Spanish, Italian—a few each day.) I would run in and there he would be in his boxers and sleeveless undershirt, shaving. Big, clean-smelling, shoulders soldier straight. He was always glad to see me, but not as glad as I was to be there. "My little Salita!" he would say. The day just started out best when I was there. He'd talk to me and give me a "button nose" (a shaving cream dollop on the tip of the nose) and tell me (if he were sad for me because he was going away on a medical lecture trip) that he just couldn't stand leaving me behind and he would like best to put some "poof powder" on me so I'd shrink and he could put me in his coat pocket and take me along. How I wished he could!

❀❀ ❀❀ ❀❀ ❀❀

Why are things always so overwhelming and cause such anxiety before you tackle them and then when you take action, launch a plan and face the problem, as bad as it may be, you seem to feel better? I was so discombobulated by the idea of moving Mother out of this house she loves that I was on an emotional roller coaster. Now that I am back home things are unfolding one step at a time and it is going, somehow, to be okay.

When the plane touched down in Memphis earlier today, Jane was waiting to whisk me away to a meeting with the powers that be at the assisted living Taj Mahal, The Gardens. Allen and Anne and their families have been on the daily local front line for so long that Jane and I have asked for the assignment of researching the options for Mother's move and making it a reality. We're glad for the chance to do it, after all that they have done week in and week out while we are living out of town, and to do it as a team. We do make a good team and we both want a hand to hold through all of this. The meeting was extremely helpful. We asked what hints the group of assisted living staff could offer from their expertise and years of experience. They said number one was to be adaptable and not to react from our own point of view, but to try and see things through **her** changed eyes. It was good advice. We are organizing as we imagine her needs to be, when really she may be a lot more ready for this new interaction than we think. She may react in some totally unpredictable way. The place and its people really do give me such a positive feeling. I told Melanie, the head of the dementia section that Mother will be in, that I felt about her the sort of instant love and dependence I felt about the nurse assigned to me during labor and childbirth. Somehow if Melanie were around it would all work out. I just knew it—though I'd never even seen her before.

❈❈ ❈❈ ❈❈ ❈❈

The birds with those same songs and conversations I have been hearing always here, that long lonesome train whistle and the clickety-clack of the train rushing, the breeze rustling all the dry leaves on the big oaks outside, sounds of people talking in the kitchen and going up and down the stairs, the cold sharp, but nice, winter breeze that came in through the windows in my old back bedroom where I was trying to air out the room after the night nurses had been smoking in there. All these things felt good as I was lying down for a catnap. I was so aware of it all. What is the line? "Drink me like your last sip of wine." That was how I felt lying there in the late afternoon's last light. Aware. Glad I'd loved it all along the way. Glad I'd stopped to feel this way now and times before. More at home than I thought I would have been with the knowledge that the countdown has started. I slept like a baby.

❈❈ ❈❈ ❈❈ ❈❈

My memories are so alive tonight. Full of growing up in this house, tying me to it. Flitting through my head. Grandmother living with us and being part of our every day. Grandmother sewing, calling out spelling words after dinner, and making us the "from scratch" cake of our choice each birthday.

Grandmother calling everyone in the whole family "Nathaniel" during the years when she could no longer remember our names—and her firstborn Nathaniel lived six states away! Daddy telling pirate stories at bedtime while we snuggled up against him. Mother saying, " Your father is only on thirty boards that meet one night a month!" Mother, the lady behind the scenes, keeping everything running smoothly. Sharp and creative, living her motto of, "Anything worth doing is worth doing well." Mother getting right down on the floor with us to play "Pick-up Sticks" or "Double Solitaire." The two of them really loved each other and children and had four of us. As I look at the photograph Daddy took to war of Mother with Allen and Jane, so small beside her, I feel how unbelievably hard it must have been for him to leave and for them to watch him go. I was the baby they had to celebrate when he came back to them at last after the war. Anne was born years later when they just wanted another child so badly after all. I was eight when Mother was expecting her and she was seven full months pregnant before I noticed something was happening. I asked Mother and she said, "Oh, yes, isn't it wonderful that we are having a baby. How should we tell Daddy?" When he came home that night I was so excited! Mother, her tummy large, and I were propped up in their big bed and Daddy came upstairs to sit in his chair beside us. I said, "Daddy, Mother and I have a **big** present for you and you have to guess what it is!" Then we played "Twenty Questions." Daddy would say, "Is it something to eat?" and we would clap our hands laughing and say, "No." " Can I play with it?" "Oh, yes!" I'd say. "Does it have scales?" Mother and I would look at each other giggling and say, "We HOPE not!" Daddy played it for all it was worth. After a long, hilarious time, he "guessed" the truth with loud surprise. I was thrilled silly! Memories . . . Allen learning taxidermy and keeping a wounded red-eyed hawk he'd rescued in his bathroom . . . and later the freezer! Jane and I sleeping together every night until she married even though we had separate rooms. Playing hairdresser with Anne's beautiful long hair. All of us have grown up and married now. Allen and Anne have big families which live close by. Jane and I live far away. Our tapestry is woven with threads from all of these people. Countless threads that are pivotal to the huge connection we feel to this place of our childhood. I feel very uneasy—out of my depth—thinking how our lives may change as we move out of it . . . and what we may soon lose.

◁◇▷ ◁◇▷ ◁◇▷ ◁◇▷

The family meeting at Allen's house was just right. We were all our own selves. Each with his or her unique way of dealing. Anne intensely taking notes on her already full calendar. Allen delegating, so fair, wanting peace in the valley, ultimately responsible. Jane centered on the sofa with papers around her, organized, full of the results of our research. And me? I don't really know. I'm sure they could fill this part in for me in a skinny minute. We don't see ourselves, do we? I loved seeing it unfold and I love those people: my brother and sisters. We are bound by so much real affection and a desire to do this well. We want to keep the great feelings we have going, full of the knowledge that what Mother and Daddy have really left us is each other. I guess it doesn't get much better than that. We have heard that these turbulent times often come with some measure of conflict and we want everyone on board up front with all decisions. We all love Mother, are realistic about her new fuzziness and childlike behavior since Daddy's death a year ago, and want the best thing for her, tough as it is. The main thing is not knowing whether what we are doing really will improve her quality of life or not. Our hope (and Donovan's good idea) is to have her spend a lot of time at The Gardens and at home and go back and forth enough so that she will feel comfortable in both places and we will get an idea of how happy she could be there. We're going to test it out with a trial run tomorrow.

P.S. Late night "back scratch train" (where you sit in a line and scratch the back of the person in front of you, guaranteed for good conversation and laughs) with Anne, little Janie Sayle, Jane and me after Mother fell asleep to old lullabies (she sang right along) and a good " back tickle."

〇〇〇 〇〇〇 〇〇〇 〇〇〇

The events are tumbling one over the other so fast that I can't keep up. I'm feeling so many different things all at once. Anyway—where to start? Icy cold runs in the morning to wake myself up, taking a love letter to a favorite cousin's house because he's inside fighting cancer and I can't go see him, home and a fast "round The Lake" walk with Jane. I was in the mood to go one more round, but she felt anxious to get started and thought we shouldn't waste time by going around again. So, we came home. We are both feeling the pressures of all this. There is going to need to be a lot of give and take over the next few weeks and we are both smart enough to sense it. Fried eggs—oh, yum! (They always remind me of home because

Mother cooked "perfect eggs" **every** morning. We'd sit down to eat and hope to finish before the carpool honked. Then we'd fly out the door, slamming it behind.) Jane and I sat on the sofa in the living room and filled out a zillion forms about Mother for the new place. We sat right there in the very room where I first saw C.D. when I was fifteen, where he kissed me the first time and where every Christmas and countless other events took place—receptions with Tony Barusso playing his music, Mother's book club meetings and Mah Jong luncheons, nights when friends would gather around the piano singing Broadway show tunes, decorating the Christmas tree while the carols blared on the Victrola and we slung icicles toward the top. Daddy watching bowl games, talking to him quietly here by the fire about the bigness of the universe and what other worlds those faraway stars might hold. Now, here we are planning Mother's move and Daddy is already gone. It all seems so jumbled up together and strange—but still somehow strangely okay.

When Mother went out to spend a little time visiting at The Gardens, Jane and I went on a major Summer Avenue thrift store blitz to look for a twin bed for Mother. We need a smaller bed and want to find one that looks like the one she's used to. The goal is to have her surrounded by familiar things so that she feels at home. It got completely hysterical when we found one in a secondhand shop and couldn't leave it to go look at any others because other buyers were eyeing it covetously. What to do? Jane took off for a quick reconnaissance of other nearby stores while I held down the fort at the junk shop. I sat on the springs of this bed we had fully put together in the middle of the floor, making phone calls on my cell phone, and waiting for her return—what a hoot! There I was in running tights, college sweatshirt, ponytail, sitting on the naked box springs of this funky bed making long distance calls in the middle of a junk store. Strange world. I couldn't believe it when I saw one of Memphis' very fanciest socialites shopping there too. Surprise! When Jane came back I was having a fine time talking to Taylor a thousand miles away at Princeton. When we went to the check-out counter an announcement came roaring over the loudspeaker: "Will the two ladies that put up the bed in the middle of the furniture area, please come back and take it down!" We just loved that.

The neatest thing though was Mother. She absolutely never batted an eye when we went out to The Gardens this noontime for lunch. She complimented her surroundings and was so gracious. When asked if she'd like to take off her coat she emphatically said, "No" several times, but a few minutes later she consented politely and basically joined right in. She greeted the other residents and patted the cute schnauzer dog that lives there. Soon Melanie announced lunchtime and called everyone to go to the dining room. Mother went happily forward with the group. Jane started forward on instinct to help her, but remembering the staff's advice, I put a hand on her arm to say, " Wait and see." Suddenly oblivious of us, Mother took Melanie's hand, walked out that door with the others, and never even looked back!

Jane and I stood in surprised silence. When our eyes caught each other's, they were full of tears.

✿✿ ✿✿ ✿✿ ✿✿

Late Tuesday night we cleared out Mother's bedside tables and dresser. It was a scream! Jane and I were rolling on the floor with silly jokes and laughter. That wonderful medicine— good hard laughter where you can't talk and your eyes water. The seriousness of all we are doing, suddenly snapping into hilarity. Such unusual items—such a rich territory: dangling coral bead earrings, the smallest pocketbook in the world, a rectal thermometer for each child, Daddy's steamy love letters and some from Mother too, Grandmother's pince-nez on a silver chain, an amazing old photograph of Mother's father suspended in the air as he actually jumped over the head of a lady standing on the beach, hand creams, soft leather gloves for much daintier hands than ours, hairpins, an ancient metal charge card from Goldsmith's in its own leather case, old birthday cards, dusting powder, ladies' fans, tiny perfume bottles all dried up, plastic gloves from the dark ages, 1920's bridge tallies, her diamond watch and pearls lost for years. I'm too sleepy—more tomorrow. (We did laugh 'til we cried over the small manila envelope boasting someone's solid gold tooth-filling inside—a gift to Mother from Daddy's identical twin brother, as his name is on the envelope with "To Jane" in his handwriting! Can you imagine? The gift for someone who has everything I should turn it in to Dave Barry for his Christmas gift list!) Jane and I haven't had this much real fun and connectedness for a long time. Another treasure.

P.S. Eight sacks of trash secretly run out to the garbage early the next AM, along with a few scary things we found in the refrigerator.

Another run this morning, solo, around The Lake. The water, a sheet of icy geometric shapes and frost turning the grass silver. The cold air in my lungs made me feel all clean inside like when you've been swimming all day. I passed the spot along the bank where C.D. and I used to sit and talk long into the night—when it wasn't too dangerous to come here at night—and when we were first really getting to know each other. I smiled. Then on around to the other side of The Lake and the spot on a brick retaining wall (now one-half submerged) where he had told me he "thought, maybe" he might love me someday. I laughed right out loud to think of that and just how lucky we'd both been that he had.

Back home I stepped inside the kitchen all hot and rich with the smell of Mother's cheery helper Brenda's big breakfast cooking and got a steaming cup of coffee. I took it out into the chilly backyard while I cooled down from the run. I walked in the foot-deep crunchy leaves, looked at Mother's garden, the bird feeders, the oaks where the hammock used to hang, the hooks all covered over by bark now. The back of that big house where I knew each window and whom it belonged to. The window sill where I used to look out late at night at the backyard silver with moonlight and write poems . . . the window where I used to smoke so I wouldn't get caught, where I thought they were fooled!

Jane and I got dressed and scooted out to make the final bed purchase (the secondhand junk shop selection won out) and get a mattress. A gal at the mattress store got all into our problem when we laid down on all the prospective mattresses, then brought in our poor pitiful bed, completely set it up in the store, and finally chose a mattress. Even with all the problem solving, we were home again by noon! It's wonderful to see so much getting done so fast. One foot in front of the other, as C.D.'s Aunt Jane says.

⚇ ⚇ ⚇ ⚇

I drove Mother to her bank later this morning and she signed some ten-year-old travelers checks we'd found during the dresser clear-out last night. The customer service rep was really nice, especially considering Mother had **no** ID with her, her signature was shaky at best, and half the checks were supposed to be signed by Daddy! When she hesitated and looked as though she might not be able to do it, I held Mother's hand, looked straight at the rep and said, "How is **your** mother?" Our eyes locked together for a few pregnant moments, then she looked down, and began processing the checks. We never mentioned those signatures again and she didn't either!

The sad part of our mission was going to buy pastries and a blossom-covered orchid for our sick cousin. Mother seemed to understand that he was sick and she wanted very much to do something for him. She was full of jumbled talk about our Irish Phillips relatives, where they had lived, what she knew of their past lives. When we dropped the gifts off at their house she very slowly and carefully signed the card "MISS Jane Hughes." Even sixty-plus years of marriage are beginning to slip away.

We took Mother out for activity time at The Gardens again today. She was so happy to be there. Kept saying how lovely everything was. Jane and I made a beeline to Home Depot to get all the things to finish the bed. It turned out that we needed about sixty dollars worth of stuff and a night of work to get a twenty-four dollar antique bed from a junk shop up to snuff. We did have the good luck to run into a Santa Claus-looking man complete with beard but minus the bowl full of jelly. He really knew woodworking and took us on. We ended up brainstorming over how to raise the bed higher and solved it by adapting newel post caps as feet! Changing the long screws in them and screwing them up into the bed legs. We did the work right there at Carl's tool demo station and it was quite a job. We got the bed project worked out, but, wow! It all took forever and we were getting late to go retrieve Mother. We began to realize just how tired we were from all the running around and then staying up late—to say nothing of the emotional ups and downs, tender moments, moments of realization about the end of an era, etc. Running on empty. We need to remember to pace ourselves or we'll burn out.

We got back to The Gardens, late by fifteen minutes and I dashed in to get Mother. When I got there she had been given some cake to eat while the others had their meal served. She and another lady resident, Cary, were at a table happily chatting (though they made little sense) and Mother told me she didn't want to leave, why didn't I just pull up a chair and stay? This kept on in gentle persuasion as basically she was perfectly content there and not up for any more activity. I only got her to come by saying she had a "dinner engagement." She took a good while assuring herself that Cary would be happy until she got back. She gave her several crackers carefully balancing them on top of each other in a teetering tower and rearranging the vegetables on Cary's plate in nice new patterns—all the while Cary in a bizarre outfit and red cap was parroting "that's nice," "okay," "that's fine," "sure," until Mother walked away smiling, a smear of whipped cream on her left cuff. It is amazing how souls find and reach out to solace each other even in these muddled states. Mother walked out graciously pausing and saying good-bye to everyone she passed as though they were all old friends, apologizing that she had to go and saying she'd be right back! Saying, "People are waiting to greet us." Who would have thought?

⟨⟩ ⟨⟩ ⟨⟩ ⟨⟩

Tired as we were, we put together a nice but quick dinner and watched the end of "Cinderella" with Mother on the little VCR we had given her. She was tired out and headed right up to bed. Jane and I collapsed in the den—making lists, brainstorming on the move and soaking in these amazing days. The lights were hurting my eyes so we turned them down and lit the big silver five-pronged candelabra. The long tapers flickering gave just the extravagant lighting we needed to get into the real feel of these fleeting momentous moments. There in the half-light we sipped (wine for her, bourbon for me) and made ourselves buckle down and finalize lists for the last meeting with The Gardens' business manager in the morning. Anne had come over today and found the social security card which had gone missing—so now we are all set for the "interview." We filled out the sheet of special info about Mother. "She's very cold-natured, likes to play the piano but doesn't remember the songs, is happy spending hours outside picking up leaves one by one." We omitted the fact that, for some reason, she has begun to snitch silverware!

Just as we were fading off to bed we realized that if we didn't do the first step in the repair of the bed and let it dry overnight, we'd not be able to have it done by the move-in deadline. Well, guess what that led to—yep, a second wind. By the time Jane and I had changed into our grubbies, gotten cardboard up on the kitchen counters to protect them, and the bed pieces laid out to work on, we were in a hilarious gig. The time flew by with so much good healthy laughing and joking. Quipping and howling over each other's dumb one-liners, we Murphy-oiled and rubbed and stained and sanded and did way more than we had ever intended to. The night just took on a life of its own. Besides the bonding fun it ended up being, the bed ended up looking absolutely super. It way outdid our expectations.

We finally did crash into bed about midnight—tired to say the least, but very happy. I admit we locked our door so Mother wouldn't come get in bed with us at four AM again. We are just too tired.

⚬⚬ ⚬⚬ ⚬⚬ ⚬⚬

On and off all night I heard the rain coming down. Is there any better sleeping than rainy nights? It is all so cozy and warm up under those covers. I slept on Mother's side this time. The depression in the mattress is just Mother's size—made over many years and about one-half as deep as the real crater on Daddy's side. It never hit me before that there are two craters. I think C.D. and I sleep so tangled up each night that there'll be just one giant one in the middle for us. I love the creaks of this old bed—it's comforting after so many years of familiarity—sort of like the rain.

My thoughts roam as I lie here. I can't help thinking how lucky we have been with Mother, the all-important timing of her move, and her attitude about everything. They say that old age is the hardest test of a person's life and from what I've seen I'd say that was pretty right on. The tough thing is that no matter how great a person you are, how strong-willed or determined to do it with grace, old age just creeps up on you and you become, one way or another, all outside of your control. There was no one nobler and finer than our father, but at the end he was very angry that life was shutting down for him before he was ready, and, though I had many good moments I'll treasure with him, sometimes he really was a bear. He would never have chosen that. On the other hand, here is Mother, who has been so accomplished and achievement-oriented, who has controlled this household and all of us with a velvet glove for years. Now she has turned aside and become malleable and adaptable. She did get very angry when we had to take her checkbook away, but after she wrote a check to a passing yardman for two thousand dollars for cutting the grass one time, we had no choice. She finally accepted it and moved on. She also had some real trouble when Daddy quit driving and decided to sell his car. Donovan and Ellen bought it and Mother still had her car, but somehow she just couldn't get that straight. For years, every time she passed the photograph of this beloved grandson and his wife that she had put on the refrigerator she would shake her head resignedly and say, "There are the people who stole my car."

She lives most of the time, however, in a positive and cheerful frame of mind. It really comes across in her daily phone conversations with me. Well, I call them conversations, but really they are more like an intricate game of Charades. Often her words get mixed up and don't come out right. Over time we have all learned how to read between jumbled words and come up with the gist. "Those things are falling" usually is about the leaves in the yard, a very popular subject as she adores to be outside picking them up. (It's ironic, but I really think those hours in the yard have given her great mental and physical health, a nice escape and a battery recharge physically.) "Our boys" means my father, the great love of her life, and his identical twin brother. (I don't believe she has spoken Daddy's name since the day he died. That day she shocked me by looking up at me serenely and saying, "A soldier or a sailor died here today.") She lowers her voice, using the whisper we all remember as the tone in which she used to tell Daddy of our misdeeds when he came home at night and talks about "these people" or "somebody is here." That means the nurses she has around the clock and it sounds as though she doesn't approve somehow, though she enjoys her daily outings with Brenda, her mainstay, and is mostly gracious to them all.

I don't think we realized until Daddy died just how mixed up Mother had become. They somehow propped each other up and were both clearer together. Once he was gone, it was like she turned off a little switch inside herself. She didn't really want to see life as it was now. After months of Daddy's heart failure and around the clock nurses, he gradually became weaker and quietly died with Mother holding his hand. That afternoon Mother was actually heard sadly telling a dear friend that came to comfort her, "You know, they never told me he was sick." Reality slowly began to dawn on us then.

What I love is that as mixed up as she is, she is still feeding my spirit. She is still showing me the way. Between the lines and sentences that don't make sense, encouragement ekes out. "We'll just take one day at a time." "I'll be right here waiting when you come and we'll have everything we need." "I'm just doing fine and not worrying about it." One of her best gifts has been the green sofa. For a long time, every day when I called her, she would tell me about the green sofa. She was very proud of herself because whenever there was anything around that she didn't know what to do about, she'd say matter-of-factly, "I just put it behind the green sofa"—the quilt pieces, the broken music box, her little stuffed monkey puppet, pictures, books, momentos, sewing projects—who knows what? After about a month of this nonsense, I couldn't wait to get home to see that sofa. And when I did, nothing was behind it! I was shocked. It was all imagination. From that day on if I have a thorny problem to solve and it's not quite ripe for a solution, I tell C.D., " I'm just going to put it behind the green sofa." He understands perfectly. It gives me great peace of mind.

Somehow, even through the fuzziness she is still giving. She is still loving. She is still lighting the way for me yet again. Teaching me how to walk this walk. Her voice lights up and she says, "Is this you, Sally?" and in those few words the rest falls away. I hear her love and that gift is enough.

Things were so different for C.D.'s mother when she came to live with us. How I loved Maggie! We had always enjoyed each other. She was beautiful, strong, and avant-garde. She was so accepting of me. In my mind, she was really the first adult not to treat me as a child. She was very happy when we asked her to come live with us and she was determined "never to be a burden." How differently it all turned out—all outside of her control. At first she was just more and more childlike—her favorite activity became watching *Sesame Street* each day with Taylor. Soon, however, she became more and more anxious, fearful and paranoid as her mind deteriorated. I'll never forget the day I was having a ladies' luncheon and we heard the dining room door squeak open. She peered around it calling, "Yoo-hoo, Yoo-hoo," and when we were suddenly hushed and she had all our attention, announced accusingly, " I know you don't care, but my house is on fire!" and stalked out, slamming the door behind.

There were all kinds of episodes with Maggie. She was a pistol. I remember one of my friends who had her mother-in-law living with her calling up and saying, "Sally, I'm mad at you." "Why on earth?" I countered. "Because your mother-in-law is full of personality and mine has me bored to tears!" That was Maggie.

She may have been referring to the hilarious, but also very poignant adventure Maggie had with the camellia bush. It all floods back to me this morning as I lie in bed listening to the rain, getting ready to get up and face the new day. It's a mixed up tale, but it says a lot about the topsy-turvy world of caretaking.

It all started when Whitney came home from a junior high slumber party one spring Saturday morning. As she came into the kitchen she asked incredulously, "What is that brassiere doing hanging on our camellia bush out front?" I looked at her puzzledly and ran outside. Sure enough, there it was, big as life! Suddenly, earlier events of the morning began to make sense.

I had awakened early to the front doorbell ringing nonstop. I came down to find an exasperated Maggie at the door in a lovely Nippon designer suit jacket without a skirt, but sporting panty-hose, and mismatched black heels. She was fussing as I hurried her inside, saying that she wanted me to come dress her. That she had tried repeatedly to get C.D. to stop his morning run and come help. (He was in training for the Boston Marathon at the time, but this particular early morning he was at the hospital seeing a patient.) She said, "I kept waving and calling him, but he just kept running by!" She was most indignant. I just brought her in and we got her all dressed and happy and I didn't think anymore of it until Whitney came home and found that brassiere—AND until I heard that the annual Ashley Hall School 3K Run had gone right past our house earlier that morning. Horrors! Maggie must have gotten tired of standing in front of the house trying to flag down a few hundred could-be C.D.s with her bra, hung it on the nearest bush, and come looking for me!

There were other amazing moments with Maggie. I give her huge credit for being the brave one, in one of her vanishing moments of awareness, to come to us and tell us it was time for her to go to a nursing home—that she just couldn't handle things well enough in our carriage house anymore, despite having a companion. It was on one of our trips for her to check out these nursing homes that she and I had one of our most telling conversations. She was telling me about something and in doing so said, "my husband, C.D." Well, the geriatric expert who had been advising us had recommended some gentle "reality adjustments" to help the senior's mind from slipping further. Things like, "This is South Carolina not Tennessee," or "It feels like Christmas, but it is really Easter." I thought this would be a good thought to readjust so I said, "You know, Walter and C.D. do have a lot in common, but Walter was your husband and C.D. is mine." "Oh, yes, of course! Walter was my husband! C.D. is yours," she confirmed and went on with her story. A moment later she was confused again when the men came into the tale. She paused. "My husband, C.D. . . . no, your . . . my . . . your husband, C.D. No, my husband, C.D.—Oh, heck! OUR husband, C.D.!" And from that day on, that's what he was.

C.D. and I were thinking, "You know, as tough as it is to solve each new Maggie problem as it comes up, at the end we'll know how best to deal with old age!" What babes we were. There are no pat solutions. It is a free fall, new every day, no two the same. As soon as you congratulate yourself for some happy resolution of one problem, the playing field changes and everything is scrambled up again. I wish there were better answers. It gets pretty overwhelming. I think I'll just put it behind the green sofa for now.

Guilt. Give guilt. The gift that keeps on giving.

I feel that guilt, even though she never gave it to me. I have it anyway and I have to try to look it in the face. The sense that it is my turn to take care of my mother at home with me the way she did for her mother and her mother did before her. It is this strongly silent example of how they made this decision and lived it out over the years and generations that speaks most loudly and eloquently. I don't remember one time when Mother ever talked about her expectations for this time of her life. To tell the truth, I think she just assumed she'd be with one of us. It has been the age-old family model and we are breaking it. That is hard even though it may be right. It is even harder because we did bring C.D.'s mother home to live with us. We were so naive and full of youthful optimism and expectations that we could solve all her problems and provide a utopian life for all of us here. It turned out to be vastly more complicated than that. Now here comes Mother who would honestly love nothing better than getting in the car with one of us at the drop of a hat and going home to live—but she's not. It is certainly not that we don't like or enjoy or love her—it is the hard fact that it just doesn't work for our world or our lives. If she were herself, mentally, and not having physical problems that make social gatherings difficult, it would be hugely different. As it is, what can we offer her that is much different from the isolation and life with attendants that she has had these last months at Headlong Hall? In a world where I was basically at home with plenty of help and family around to be there whenever I had a carpool or something, it might have worked. That is how my home was as I grew up. Someone—Mother, Grandmother, our beloved housekeeper Bernice —was home all the time. I cannot remember **ever** coming home to an empty house. Our world is different now, and I am gone a lot of the day. Our youngest, Langdon, is in school all day. I am out painting—which is my life work and my passion. I don't think for a minute Mother would want me to walk away from that to devote myself to these last "iffy" years of hers. She probably would like me to be clever enough to figure out a way to do both happily.

Increasingly, it seems that she operates on the feeling of "out of sight, out of mind." Emotional at seeing us, but forgetting us the moment we walk out the door. Allen was having a lovely visit with her recently and she always lights up to see him. In the middle of their talk, however, someone passed by her door and Mother got up mid-sentence and walked right past him out the door and got on the bus for an outing without so much as a glance! This has to make one wonder if having her at home would be really fulfilling for her or whether she is just as happy at The Gardens. I can see in a hundred ways that she is better served where she is with people who are equipped to handle all the downsides and augment all the positive possibilities. But it isn't us. If my head is so sure, then why does my heart get these twinges and why the guilt? I remember Cousin Weetie helping me once by telling me about her mother's care. She said, "Sally, No matter how much you do, it is just in the nature of the situation that you never feel it is quite enough. You have to be easy on yourself." I don't know how our generation will work out these feelings in such a rapidly changing culture of two-job families and living far from the old homeplace. I think they are inevitable feelings in our active lives. We love our parents, owe them tremendous honor and thanks for all they've given us, and now we are too busy becoming those very people they encouraged us to be. Should we stop our worlds, get off, and reinvent ourselves to take care of them for who knows how long? It is a dilemma. My head, my instincts, my heart are almost at peace with each other—but not quite. Maybe they never will be. Maybe these particular puzzle pieces just can't ever quite fit together.

⬥⬥ ⬥⬥ ⬥⬥ ⬥⬥

No run today, just one of Brenda's big hot egg breakfasts with Mother before she left for the beauty parlor. Jane and I had a final appointment at The Gardens over the last details. It looks as though my next trip back in a few weeks is when we'll move her things in on Sunday. Then that next Monday, January twenty-second, will be the first night sleeping there, with Jane and me holding our breaths in The Gardens' guest room upstairs.

We checked off last "to do's" as we drove around and did errands. Rain still pouring. When we got home, Mother looked so tired that we canceled her outing to visit The Gardens. Jane made calls to unravel financial questions while I lacquered the bed and measured items to go. We both organized her clothes to take. Sorting what she'll need, what looks nicest on her, what will stay nice looking the best. As we stood with our heads in the middle of her closet, Jane looked up at me and said, "Do you realize what we are doing?!" We stopped cold and looked at each other for a long moment.

I'm not sure that I do. It seems unreal somehow. Safety in the details. Lots of details.

All her clothes are now in Daddy's vacant closet waiting for the helpers to sew in nametags. We are using all the pretty embroidered ones she and Grandmother always sewed into our camp clothes by hand—none of those Sharpie laundry markers for her. The end of an age. It's such a small group of belongings. She will leave this house with one tiny closet of clothes. It reminded me of Anne Morrow Lindbergh's *Gift From the Sea* where she muses that at the end of one's life we are like the chambered nautilus—transparent and without belongings—purely "us."

❊❊❊ ❊❊❊ ❊❊❊ ❊❊❊

Jane waved as she drove away to head back to her home. I came in and put "Snow White" on the VCR. Mother can still somewhat understand and enjoy the old classic stories of her childhood. We cozied up on the green sofa, I with my head in her lap, and watched it. She stroked my hair and we laughed at all the funny parts and held hands. She proudly showed me the small clip hoop earring she is now wearing as a ring. She is delighted by the clever way it opens and closes.

At one point, I looked around this library full to the ceiling with great books and Mother's oil paintings, Daddy's mounted Alaskan salmon and Mississippi turkey tail, his brigadier general's hat on the shelf beside the pediatric texts he had written and that we used to peek at during slumber parties to see what was what. I soaked it in. Slowly. Very slowly. Seeing it all a bit differently from my vantage point with my head in Mother's lap and on this particular night. I wanted to memorize every inch. The family photographs, Daddy's big desk, the horse sculptures, Mother's sewing basket and tiny scissors. I felt how it was at this late date to be here like this with her and how this "heart home" would soon cease to hold me anymore.

⬤⬤ ⬤⬤ ⬤⬤ ⬤⬤

It's strange how one can love a place so much and feel a part of its spirit and still be ready to let it go. As much happiness as I have had here, there has also been real loneliness and emptiness. Adolescent doubts and insecurity, eagerly waiting for a call from a certain someone that never came, watching Daddy bury our old dogs in the back flower bed, feeling on the edge of life and being slightly misunderstood, wondering which way to go with my life, wondering if I would ever get a figure like the other girls. I think I always yearned for that thing that would make me whole, let me be a grown-up and walk away on my own life's journey. I remember at sixteen standing in the dark several winter nights after supper looking out the living room window across the front lawn and feeling painfully lonely. I thought that I would give anything to see C.D. walk across from the bridge across the way toward our house, but he was miles away at college. There was so much yearning.

The truth is that I'm passing from this part of my life, but I wouldn't have it any different. I wouldn't give up living in Charleston, or being married with my own children, or my art, or friends, to live here again. I don't want it back—I just want to appreciate and remember and soak in all I can of this huge part of my becoming. I don't want to live here, but I sure would like to take the sound of those trains home with me.

Janie Sayle came to Headlong Hall to spend the night. Anne is coming later after the art class she teaches—about ten o'clock. Janie, twelve, did homework and I put Mother to bed. It was so cold in the house (the mysterious heating control was down to sixty degrees) that Mother refused to take off the velvet warm-up suit we gave her for Christmas. You know, I really didn't blame her. I decided it just wasn't worth the battle this time to get that warm-up off and her gown on. She seems somehow weary inside tonight. Am I just imagining that some deep part of her senses and knows what this intense visiting and activity are all about? Is it her sadness or my guilt that, as irrational as it is, compels me to make it all better for her and I can't?

I did get her to have a successful trip to wash up for bedtime and then said, "Now, let's brush our teeth." She said a flat and emphatic, "No. I don't want to brush my teeth. I will not brush my teeth." When I mentioned her wanting to smell fresh, she adamantly refused again. After another try, I said, "Okay, Let's don't. Let's fold this towel instead." As I began to fold, I casually handed Mother her toothbrush with the Colgate on it to hold and she turned seamlessly and did a wonderfully thorough job of brushing her teeth. It is a new world. And I am learning fast! Diversion is my new favorite word.

The irony is that it was Mother herself who taught us all this ideal technique of using diversion rather than confrontation to handle unruly children. Suddenly, here I am using it on her. Who is the grown-up now? I am realizing how much easier it was just to be the unruly child. Now I have to step up and be the grown-up, and I don't want to have to.

One of the best things about my trips home over the last few years has always been getting into the bed with Mother when she is going to sleep, trading back scratches (she is the all-time best—never wastes a movement and never seems to get tired of it) and singing the old lullabies and songs she still recognizes. Tonight was no different—with one twist. We started out singing, "There's a pale moon shinin' on the fields below . . . " then moved to, "Is it True what They Say about Dixie?" "Harvest Moon," "Someone's in the Kitchen with Dinah," "Good Night Ladies," and "Jesus Loves Me." The twist was the back scratch. After scratching her back, we turned over as we always do so she could do mine. I nestled down happily to enjoy it and she started scratching evenly and nicely up and down my back as she has done countless times. Next, she was happily going under my underpants elastic. I thought, well, she is my own mother and she's easing that elastic mark. Before I knew it those sweet hands were moving further down toward places that don't get scratched! She'd forgotten the lines you don't cross—those instinctual boundaries had just vanished. Up I sat with a start. "Your turn!" I gasped. She turned over contentedly, completely unaware, and before long I heard the even breathing of sleep. That is one back scratch that certainly got out of hand . . . another shift in the playing field.

Little Janie and I propped up in the big master bed and read books. It was so delicious. By the time Mother was asleep I felt like it was midnight, but in truth it was only about seven-thirty! I loved curling up with Janie—she with *Harry Potter* (I think she said, "for the third time") and I with this journal and the next book for my wonderful book club. I couldn't get into the book. I'm living too intensely my own saga just now and the book's adventures and descriptions just seemed flat to me. I liked being propped up there just like Mother and Daddy used to be in the mornings for "coffee time." That was their term for the early morning when they would have coffee in bed. They would ring the buzzer to wake us up at the other end of the house and we would trundle in all sleepy and curl up like puppies on the bed with them before we had to get up and dress for school. We would talk about the day ahead, or things in general, and just wake up together. How we used to love to be the one asked to run downstairs and get the newspaper for Daddy.

Every now and then as we read, Janie would make a comment into the silence, totally out of the blue. "I have never been able to learn how to walk through that hall without having every board squeak. I've conquered the stairs though." And later, "I had a journal too once, but I got behind in it. When I tried to catch up, there were whole chunks gone out of my life." Such wisdom from a twelve-year-old! Then into the silence, "I have a book where I write poems. I pick a subject like 'computers' or 'Bob' and I compose a poem about that." To confirm this, she recited one about Bob and then one about Jim.

Janie makes for a very interesting bedfrog.

We had both fallen asleep by the time Anne got home. I heard her loudly knocking on the back door—locked out on the scary back porch due to the cranky old lock. How MANY times that has happened to us all! I ran down and rescued her and we came on upstairs, all of the stairs creaking just as Janie had said. Then, of course, we had to talk in bed until way too late because we're never together enough and have so much to tell each other—so we did. Just as we were fading off half-awake, half-asleep, Anne said, "I love it when we talk. I can be so open. I don't have to pretend anything at all with you." I reached for her hand, and we fell asleep.

❁❁ ❁❁ ❁❁ ❁❁

I fly back to Charleston today. I had pictured this morning as a last relaxed, lazy breakfast time with Mother. Anne and Janie were off early to get her to school and Mother and I were together. As much as it should have been us puttering over the frying bacon and eggs, it was me getting my stuff back in the suitcase, answering the phone, getting dressed, finding the plane ticket. Ah, anticipation.

It was all right. We did sit down together in the library with our trays. She in the brown leather chair she likes best and I on the green sofa.

It was one of those moments when I expected to have realizations that were powerful or feel deeply the fact that this scene and moment could never come again. Instead, I felt nothing but unrest and churning. It was like all the air had gone out of the balloon of feeling and we were just there together.

Marking time. "Say something I'll never forget." Wanting to be connected, but somehow missing the mark. Wanting to say something that would pull Mother's mind to me and share some good old reliable family story or laugh together. "Do you remember when so and so did such and such?" But no. This is the hard part. This is the real letting go.

Whom are we more centered on as we grow up—other than our own little selves—than on our mother? Whom are we bound to in every way? Whom do we want to praise us? Whom do we run to in every need? We need her and that's a pull. She needs us and that's a pull. Now she doesn't feel the need anymore. She loves me . . . would give me anything, from the bronze horse lamps to her used paper napkin. But she really feels no strong pull, no need anymore. Realization swamps me. The umbilical cord is cut. I float free. My loss is enormous. But, I'm a big girl now and I have to take it. She has been teaching me all my life how to take it. From the day I was born, she has been preparing me to march to the end of the branch, look back and smile, and fly. It was her goal, but can I do it?

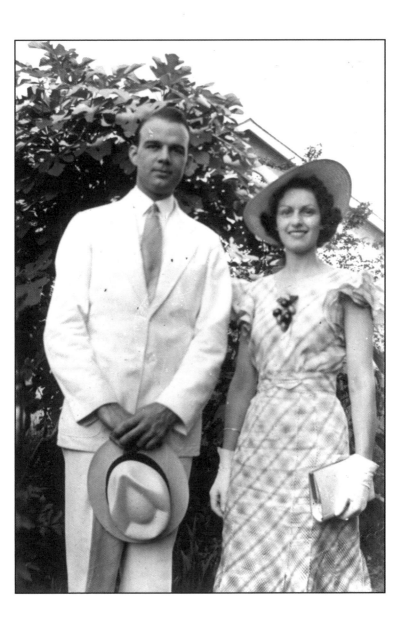

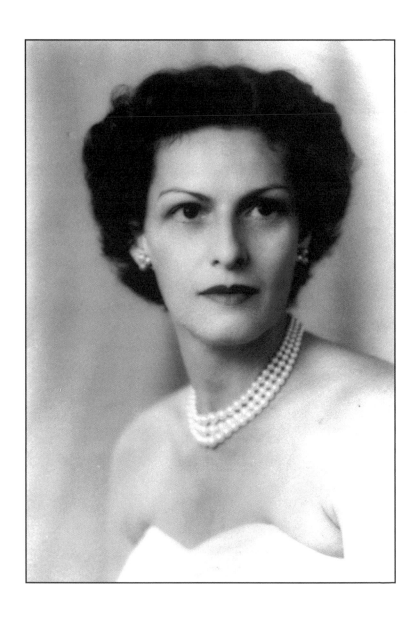

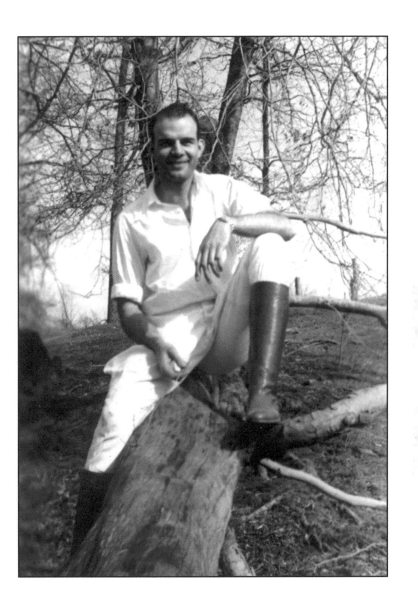

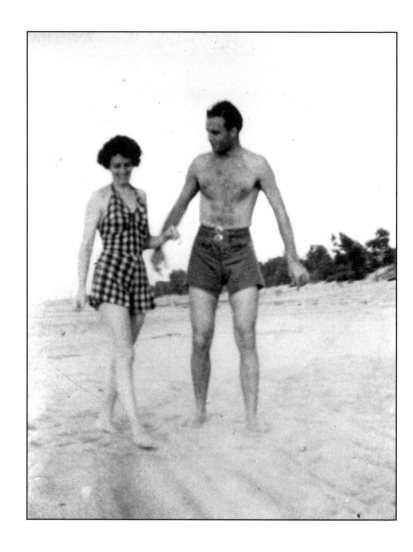

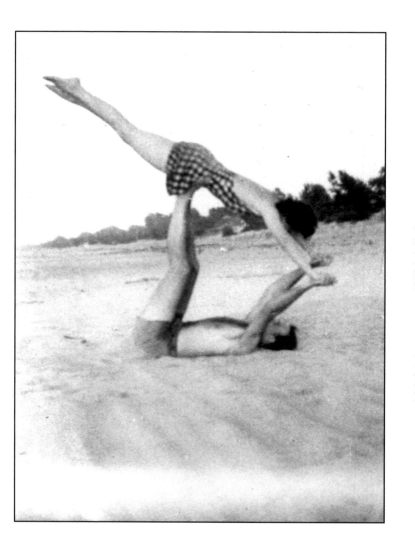

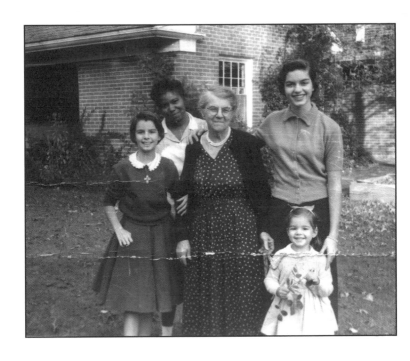

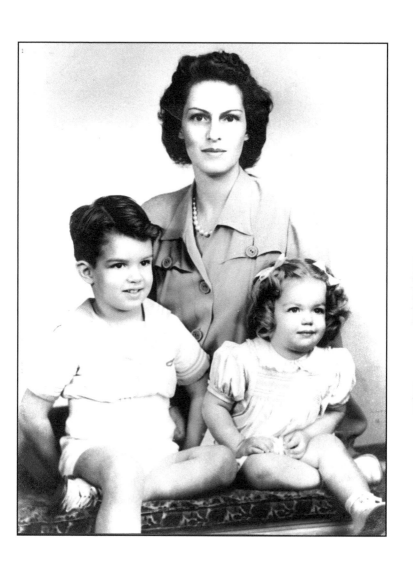

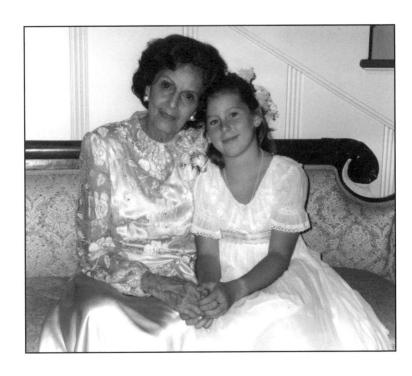

2
SECOND TRIP BACK HOME

I woke up this morning very unsettled. All is packed for my return to Memphis to actually move Mother. All the "to-do's" are done, but I feel uneasy. The odds for a major upheaval are so high. I feel almost desperate to see C.D. and feel his calming influence on me. Something to give me the quiet steady reserve to deal with whatever may come. Somehow, like a child, I irrationally think maybe he'll even tell me I can't go. But he's at the hospital for a meeting this morning. I know this restless energy and I know the best thing for it is to spin it out on some project—so I go to the attic and whirl through tasks at my desk that I have put off for months. It does help. Then Langdon breezes in between spending the night out and babysitting—such a happy spirit, such a breath of fresh air. So good through and through and so oblivious of the time-worn problems like moving mothers out of their nests. Still willing to hug a mother who needs a hug. Then the door slams and she's off. Did I hug my mother enough? I hope so. I think so.

C.D.'s hand on the door and I'm into the front hall in a flash. How those arms around me seem to fill me and renew the knowledge that everything will be all right—that we can handle anything. We cook up a big breakfast and he sees that I'm uneasy. His eyes hold mine.

"How long do we have before you leave for your plane?"

"Two hours."

"Good."

"How I love to be in Mammy's arms when it's sleepytime w-a-y d-o-w-n S-o-u-t-h . . ."

I'm back and Mother is curled up on her side of the bed getting her back scratch. (I'm skipping mine from now on!) We sing "Blue Moon," "Sleepytime Gal," "Singing in the Rain," "Darktown Strutter's Ball." I picture Mother all lithe and slim in the long organdy dresses we found in the attic. All cut on the bias, of course, with side plaquets, big ruffled scoop neck and starched flounce around the bottom. I remember being little and watching them get all dressed up to go to a ball. Daddy, looking grand in his tuxedo, asked expansively, "Sally, how would you like to go to the ball and dance with Daddy?" "Oh, no," I replied, looking at Mother in her fancy satin gown, "I want to go to the ball and dance with Mother!" I can picture her when they were younger with Daddy, elegant in his tux, dancing to the big band swing music at the Skyway Lounge on the Peabody Hotel's roof like their crowd used to do. Cabaret tables. Cigarette girls. Painted ceiling and soft lights. Rooftop promenade. Laughter. Full moon shining on the Mississippi River. Daddy with his ivory cigarette holder. Skirts whirling. Classic. No one with pierced earrings. Small evening bags with tiny compacts. Calling card cases. Gloves. Hair swept off their faces.

The last time I was up in the attic, I tried on one of those organdy gowns—the blue one made of dotted Swiss and felt triumphant I could even get it over my head and pulled down. Forget trying to snap up all those tiny snaps. She was so straight and girlish then—so full of life. Now she is slightly bent, eighty-nine, and, miraculously, still full of life!

Today was all in a fog. Everything went like clockwork, just as it was planned. Anne and Allen came. The four of us waited until Mother had finished breakfast and gone on her daily drive—and then, swoosh! Down on the house we came, all action and organization, Jim arriving to help carry the heavy pieces, packing things we'd planned to take in the cars for the move out to The Gardens. Lots of bustle and energy.

I got to ride out with Allen, which I always love. We had a good talk about balance and these decisions we're now caught up in. Timing and how important that is in Mother's move. Waiting to find the moment when she was confused enough to adapt without being upset, yet not too confused to make a life there and benefit from the interaction they have to offer her. How steady and strong he has been throughout this confusing time. Always ready to think the best of us all.

The room came together in a snap. All the measuring and planning Jane and I had done really paid off. We had just the right pieces and tools to get everything into place. Before we knew it, we had an amazingly charming little nest for her.

After all the action of the day, we came back home to have family lunch with her. All of us—all the ages, around the dining room table. Telling tales. Catching up. Her great-grandson, Will, at one-and-a-half, smiling and pulling up to look out of the French windows as so many of us have done. Mother loves to tell how she told the architect that she wanted windows low enough so that the babies could look out and the dogs could look in.

When the group faded, Mother, Jane, and I sat down and

did some puzzles at the little table by the kitchen window. They were simple ones, about twenty-five pieces, and big shapes. Something she could have some success doing with us steering her toward the right fit. Just what we wanted. We laughed and joked and high-fived each other. We had good hard laughs. Really connecting. It felt so good. We'd finish one and say, "Let's do just one more!" It is her last afternoon in this house.

☉ ☉ ☉ ☉

In the rosy sun of late afternoon we walked around The Lake together. How many times have we all done that? She does love seeing those ducks and geese! Whenever she'd say, "Let's go here," or "That path is muddy, let's go there," we would follow her lead, both Jane and I sensing that she was still in control and soon that would be changing. We wanted to do whatever she wanted to do.

We feasted in the dining room by candlelight. The Last Supper. Time is flying.

"Cinderella," tried and true, was our movie choice again tonight. Mother sat between us on the green sofa and we were snuggled up under one of the warm afghans Irma Buckingham made for Mother forever ago. Mother was placidly holding a glass of orange juice in her hand and Jane and I were both eager for her to drink it up—Jane, because we'd put her nightly Tylenol PM ground up in it and I, for that reason as well, and because I was dying to put my head in Mother's lap while we watched the movie and her glass was there instead. About the time Cinderella went to the ball, my head was in her lap and we finished out the movie in that special cozy way. We were just as delighted as always that the glass slipper really does fit and those wicked stepsisters are foiled again. Dreams really can come true. I hope ours for a happy move do. I think Mother's dreams have for her whole life. That feels good to know—to say. What more could she want than what she got? Born into a wonderful family, true love, a meaningful productive life, four healthy children that grew up respecting and loving her and still do, long years of good health and a lot of laughter. May we all be so lucky!

❧❧ ❧❧ ❧❧ ❧❧

This morning has been like a dream. One where I feel like I am walking in slow motion and each frame of the action is clear and defined.

Cold, icy walk with Marily and Jane at dawn, and then I jog The Lake by myself, feeling the morning sun on my face and the crunch of frozen grass under my feet. My lungs cold and clear, my footsteps thudding—leaping the gnarly roots close by the bank—padding across the wooden bridge. **I am so alive**. I am still so many years from Mother's time. Mortality sending me an adrenalin rush of realization that my time is **now** and that it doesn't last forever. It is only right to exult in that potential and savor it to the hilt—to feel hungry for life. To celebrate the amazing fact of being alive to see and feel and hear, to have a friend, to laugh, to think, to be connected. To be exhilarated by this free gift of life that we have each been given. Like when I was in high school and college and sometimes I felt as though I would burst with the joy of just being alive—just walking down the street, for no reason at all. Where does that come from? Is it in my DNA? Did my parents give it to me? I hope everybody in the world feels that way sometime. I'd like to bottle it and pass it out for free.

The perfect eggs, the perfect bacon, Mother redoing one of the little puzzles from yesterday. Working so studiously over something so simple to her just a few years back, but enjoying it. This, the same clever lady that our housekeeper Bernice always bragged on by saying, "Give Miss Jane a string and a brick and she can fix anything!"

Jane went ahead to do a little pre-arrival setting up and I realized that we were down to only thirty minutes with her in that house. What is amazing when I think of it, is how much life was crammed into that brief time.

Brenda was dressing Mother's hair, so I sat on a stool at Mother's feet and read nursery rhymes upside down in a book on her lap so she could see the pictures. We both knew most of the words—Mother remembering much more than usual—seeming especially alive this morning. We laughed uproariously at some of the old endings. We'd look up from the book and into each other's eyes and burst out laughing— "All fall down!" "Licked the platter clean!" "Georgie Porgie ran away." It was so warm and cozy and I was glad that dear Brenda was there, part of our special circle of love.

As I was getting up, Mother, feeling playful, pulled me back down into her lap and began to rock me and sing, "Rock-a-bye baby in the treetops . . . " Arms entwined, boisterous and happy we were. When we came to "Down will come cradle, baby and all," she opened her legs and dumped me on the floor! I knew what was coming because she always loved that part best. We were full on laughing then, she was feeling **so sassy.** A smile is on my face as I think of it now.

_____

I felt the clock ticking. We strolled hand in hand through the living room and she pointed out her treasures as she likes to do. We looked out those lovely French doors across the patio to the sunlight soaking the trees and her flower beds she has worked in so. She walked to the piano, oh, wonder of wonders, and ever so softly began to play. "Would you like me to play?" she looked up sweetly, amiably asked—ready at a word to stop if I should not want her to continue. She was just happy to do whatever I thought best. Amazing. And the music so sweet and soft had unity and tune—probably some harmony from deep within her days of playing—like a tattered piece of a battle flag that still held on.

I sat beside her as still as a mouse and felt so peaceful. I wondered if Daddy was listening. I wondered at the beauty and fullness of each phase and each passage of our lives, at this excruciatingly beautiful thing called life. What is that line from *The Sound of Music?*— "When God closes a door, he always opens a window." Somehow we adapt and have what we need for what comes next.

❈❈ ❈❈ ❈❈ ❈❈

How we dreaded those first steps into Mother's new rooms. We had all looked at this moment from every angle—how best to have it be happy. Talking to her beforehand would have been like reasoning with a small child—upsetting and ineffective. Jane said it best when she said, "If you ask a small child if they want to go to bed, they will probably say 'No.' " The same holds for Mother. Our hope was that by surrounding her with things she loves, she would focus on those and feel at home. Our plan was to have her spend a lot of time at The

Gardens and at home and go back and forth enough so that she felt comfortable in both places. It seems to have worked so far. She walked in and looked at her oil paintings and her familiar furnishings without saying a word. She fingered all the little touchstones she was used to seeing on her dresser—the china rose, the Italian leather box with her name in gold, the antique doily, the photographs—and was seriously curious, but not ruffled. "Don't you find it peculiar that this portrait of me is here?" she asked. We just said how lovely it was. Other than that, she really seemed an example, again, of feeling that what was out of sight, was out of mind, with no remembrance of Headlong Hall holding these objects for the past fifty-odd years until today. Before long some residents came by and she was proudly receiving compliments on her paintings and showing them off enthusiastically.

Her innate trust of her world and of us and her innate bravery were so clear to me in those minutes. I was choked up and I looked at her through a veil of tears as she took the hit.

Dealing with the "peculiarness" of what was somehow out of the twilight zone—all of her things in a foreign place and Jane and I hanging up our coats in a closet full of her clothes. She looked around and then settled in and accepted that it must somehow be okay. The foundation for the ability to do that was probably laid back in her own loving and secure childhood where she was able to trust in the world as a basically good and happy place. How thankful I was for that trust now! At some level I believe she knows things are changed and how moving it was to see that brave little spirit walk into a totally new life with equanimity. I was just proud to know her.

How she teaches us step by step to walk this walk even from beyond her fog. I cannot think of that moment even now without fierce pride and love and tears that take me by surprise with their suddenness.

3
AFTER THE MOVE

It is amazing how fast things can change. From total absorption in Mother and giving her our undivided attention, to being told that we needed to leave her be to have a chance to adjust and get comfortable with her new surroundings. I think we felt a bit like new mothers who leave that precious baby for the first time at Mother's Day Out.

Mother walked off happily to go on a drive with the group as though Jane and I weren't even there. We turned and headed for the car like a couple of zombies . . . Talk about shell shock. We couldn't believe that the hurdle had been met and passed without a major upheaval! We had been dreading the possibilities of her reaction for months. I felt that I had just narrowly missed having a car wreck. It was a world altering change for her, and really for us too, because that home has always had her there welcoming us whenever we walked in the door. Bringing friends, then dates, then husbands and children over our lives. Always a cozy bed for you and yours, animated conversation, warm acceptance. That ends tonight. The house is still there, but the heart has gone.

In true Hughes fashion, we headed back to Headlong Hall slowly turning our thoughts to what comes next. We have been so focused on Mother's gentle entry into a new phase of life that we haven't really looked beyond that. That good amount of energy that we have all got stored up and an open day ahead of us had us sorting and cleaning all day. A big dose of action is such a healthy thing!

It is really scary how fast a house that holds the accumulations of a lifetime and treasures filtered down from a large and diverse family can be culled down to the basics. Boxes of categories fill up fast—Daddy's old pipes, kid gloves, years of family photos, ancient bifocals in leather cases with purple lining, satin lingerie cases, clocks, unidentified keys, wonderful old children's toys, exotic inlaid boxes, crystal dresser jars, a lovely handle with a chamois cover for buffing fingernails, handkerchiefs with so much lace around the edges that they are totally useless for their intended purpose, jewelry, including a tiny folded wax paper with, "Is this the diamond from my old ring?" in Mother's hand and no diamond inside (this found in a little drawer of pencils in Grandfather's desk!). Then there is the BIG box that says "Goodwill" in Magic Marker on the side. It's filling fast with vases, blankets we never liked, clothes, TV tables, sheets with floral prints from the '60s, hats, on and on—and next to that an even bigger one marked "Trash." These boxes fill up faster than they can be carried out and come back in again. Medicines from years ago, old lipsticks, plastic bags, rugs, irons that don't work, chipped vases, dishcloths, papers, paper Mexican flowers, clothes the Goodwill doesn't want, an old fake Christmas wreath, magazines, incomplete decks of playing cards, string, potting pots, once usable garden tools, clothespins and line. And then there's the "Recycling" bin. I wish I could see the faces of the recycling collectors when they come next—tons of old pickle jars, old florist's containers mixed in with plastic milk cartons. There were lots of old, but not charming, brown bottles from which we dumped out the most astonishing assortment of contents. I'm amazed the drain didn't start to sizzle and smoke with the concoction! Some of them had the old paper labels glued on by hand from our long gone corner drugstore, Bobbit-Doer. (How I remember the thrill of Mother saying it was okay for me to stop by there on the way home from first grade each day and get an ice cream cone—a monumental nickel each it cost us.) Allen and I agreed we had to save the one old milk bottle from the days when each morning we'd open the back door to get the fresh milk the milkman had delivered at dawn. Thick cream covering the top under the foil cover. Daddy would have the cream in his coffee. Who ever heard of low-fat then?

▨▧ ▨▧ ▨▧ ▨▧

The day turned into late afternoon in a flash. Before we realized it, Jane and I were rushed to throw some dinner together for ourselves, put it in a sack to eat once we had put Mother to sleep, throw some clothes in our suitcases for spending the night, and sprint out to Mother's new emporium.

She lit up when she saw us come in and said, "Oh, you're here!" But she basically seemed relaxed and content. We learned from the assistants that she had had a good day and had begun to make some friends, which was music to our ears. After chatting awhile, we said, "Well, let's go to bed now. I'll put my nightgown on and we'll put yours on too." She was perfectly willing. While Jane went to settle some bags upstairs in the guest room where we were to spend the night, Mother and I put on our gowns, brushed teeth, and pulled back the covers on the pretty little resurrected bed. We were snug in that tiny bed together before I would have thought it possible.

I must say I did wonder at first if the bed would prove sturdy enough to hold both of us, but it, like Mother, pulled through like a champ.

Lights low, I began singing. "There's a pale moon shining on the fields below . . . " and there she was chiming in and singing along just like always. What a moment! I shut my eyes and held on to it. It just seemed impossible that so much had happened so fast and here we were—same nighties, same songs, same us—all under a totally different roof. Life going on. The river never never stopping, just flowing over new terrain. Adapting itself. Adapting herself.

It turned out to be a thirty-song night instead of the usual five- or six-song night. Mother was definitely stirred up—restless. Her fingers moving, tapping, certainly not sleepy. As I rubbed her neck I would ask, "Are you getting sort of sleepy?"

"No, not really."

We joined together to do our favorite old soft lullabies that she has sung to us for so long. When she still wasn't tired, we did all the old big band favorites I could remember. When she was still wide-eyed, we tried my old camp songs. When that didn't work, I sang my friends' camp songs they'd taught me from their camps. We even threw in her old favorite "Ab-dull-a-bull-bull-a-mere." Burl Ives finally did the trick. "Story of the Grey Goose," "I Had a Goat, His Name was Jim," "Mr. Rabbit, Mr. Rabbit." Appropriately, "Amazing Grace" was last. She was softly breathing now. I enjoyed the silence. At one point in the singing rounds, Mother had turned toward me and said in her jumbled, almost clear way that we should really spend more time working on our singing because we could be quite good. The idea was that somehow we could do well and get ahead in the world doing it. She made the point that we could make something of ourselves and not just "goof off" during our spare time.

Always, forever teaching—encouraging us to be all that we can be. Feeding the drive to use our God-given talents to the fullest—which was in our parents' genes and which has been passed on to us to pass on again. That wonderful circle again.

I stayed a few more minutes just being thankful. Enjoying her, warm against me. Just trying to feel all that had happened to her and us in these last few hours. Monumental change for all of us. Wondering how hard it would be to give it, if you never got it. I can undress my mother and put her in a nightgown and we play the same silly games we delighted in when we were little and she was big—saying peek-a-boo when her head comes through the neck. It is natural to snuggle with her in the bed when she has put us to bed that way a thousand times. The songs are all from her. What do people do that do not have this beautiful pattern to follow? These instincts planted long ago with no thought of how they might one day play out, changing hands and generations. How do people learn this language if they were never given these ministerings? I can't imagine how the scenario would be then. Much harder, I would think. Our mother touched and hugged us—so it is easy to touch and hug her. Our mother was always there for us and did whatever it took to do what she thought was right for us. So, it is perfectly natural to be there for her and we are, to a person, willing to do whatever it takes to do right by her. When you have gotten it, your instincts are all in place to give it. I wish people who have not been lucky enough to be given these loving patterns could stand in my shoes for awhile and feel what this growing up was like. That it might help them somehow be able to give this way too, even if they are starting from a different and more difficult place. Transition makers. A hard but very beautiful thing to be. Breaking an old cycle and starting a better, warmer one from scratch.

⚬⚬ ⚬⚬ ⚬⚬ ⚬⚬

I must admit Jane and I were pretty exhausted. Mostly from passing through such an emotional day—one we had hardly dared hope would go so well. The day flew by partly because we are good at diving into projects and partly because it helped to divert us from worrying about Mother. When I slipped out into the hall in my robe and slippers, Jane was sitting there Indian style against the door waiting to see if I needed "spelling" with Mother. She was reading one of those nutty romantic histories Mother has liked so the last years. Little mini-brain vacations we all partake of when we're home . . . and there has certainly been a need for healthy mini-brain vacations along this sometimes overwhelming path.

We went up to our quarters in the guest suite and settled in. It was almost nine o'clock. We realized how famished we were. Even more important was the realization that we had somehow gotten out the door with a nice bottle of wine and no corkscrew. There was no question of accepting the absence of a corkscrew without a fight. We wanted a celebration! When no corkscrew could be unearthed from the kitchens below, Jane became most resourceful. First we tried a large screw she had found in the exercise room. Then we tried a curtain hook! The real moment of genius came when she thought a moment, got out her Chapstick, lined it up carefully with the cork, and hammered it in with her shoe. Voila! Vino! Laughter—again, the perfect relief.

We laid out the quilt we had brought for Mother's bed on the floor so we could have a picnic. The dinner had suffered a good bit from the long delay between cooking and eating, but we knew that hunger would make a good sauce. Out of the sack came Jane's container of now cold soup and I hope I long remember her cry of delight when she remembered that she had put once hot toast in there with it. Christmas morning had nothing on this happy discovery. The only problem was that we'd also forgotten a spoon. Aha! Another chance to solve the unsolvable and we do love solving puzzles! We were on a roll and loving it. After running through a few funny options, I suddenly realized that the large end of my celery stick looked a whole lot like one of those china Oriental spoons. More laughter. Jane graciously accepted the largest celery stalk and the meal was on. We feasted flamboyantly on such delicacies as cold soup and crumbled toast with a great deal of toasting out of plastic bathroom cups. We've certainly been to finer dinner parties, but not one that was more hilarious than this one!

We fell into bed tired from laughing and from the day's emotions and ready to sleep like logs. Imagine my surprise when I felt something as I put my legs between the sheets and pulled out a pair of someone else's prescription eye glasses! The last occupant of the guest suite, no doubt. We started laughing all over again. How could this be? Our sides hurt. What was going to happen next? We didn't even care. I tossed the glasses off the bed and we were out like lights.

We were so eager to see how things had gone for Mother during the night! We waited like anxious suitors for the exact time we had been told we could come see her. When we got down for coffee at the appointed time, we learned that all had gone beautifully. She was up, had bathed and dressed, and eaten a hearty breakfast. Music to our ears.

We took a pretty little tray with coffee and fixings into her room for a "tea party." How nice and sunny the room and Mother looked. She was animated and smiling, sitting up in the armchair looking out into the garden. I sat cross-legged on the end of our now favorite bed and poured us all cups. It was very cozy. Mother enjoyed the undivided attention. Melanie and her helpers dropped in on and off to say hello and talk about her paintings. At one point she told them, "You know, it is so wonderful that these paintings I did so long ago happened to end up here on these walls after all this time. I haven't seen them in years!" Jane and I silently rolled our eyes at each other.

Mother sang some nursery rhymes with us as we looked through her pretty book together. She seems to remember songs better than how to speak. I wonder why. It is another way for us to connect and I am just happy for any way I can to do that.

She turned without a backward glance and walked out of the room when activity time came. We still can't get used to this "out of sight, out of mind," but it is for real. Jane and I left for Headlong Hall to meet Anne and whoever had a yen to sort and chuck out.

Another full day. Another night putting Mother to sleep. Another full day. Another visit to love on Mother. So the new circle or maybe it is still a part of the old one—goes rolling steadily on.

We'll never be quite the same. Not one of us. Will we be more? A resounding "Yes!" to that. Even for Mother whose material world has just shrunk from a mighty plenty to the size of a pea. She has this last good chance to connect to people and have warm people-filled days in a supportive place with kindhearted helpers.

And for us? Oh, yes. These days have stretched us all and tested us all. We've been asked to reach down and pull up the best within us as we hold hands and walk wherever this takes us. A walk, we have all heard, that is not easy on families, even close ones. We've been trying to keep our eye on the goal and let the little, petty things fall away. We have honestly tried to see each decision through the eyes of the others, realizing that we each have a right to our own point of view and that there usually is no clear "only" way things have got to be. Everyone has had a chance to speak, even if they haven't always taken it. Everyone has had a turn listening. Still, there have been imperfect times. As a family, we are averse to conflict and pass through those sticky times and act as if they never really happened. Some people might think every grievance is healthier aired out, but we avoid that unpleasantness and move on. It is our way of coping in an imperfect world and it has worked for us as it might not work for others. We have made an effort to be easy on each other and tough on the problems, even though we have sometimes failed. The key is that we are trying. We are the living fruit of what she hoped for us as a close family.

Through teaching us how to get along all these years, she has given us each other. The best part is that we really like what we got! When she is no longer here to stand beside us, we will still have each other for as long as the journey lasts. That comforts me hugely.

May the circle be unbroken.

⬡⬡ ⬡⬡ ⬡⬡ ⬡⬡

"Oh, sure," I hear myself say. "How unreal does this Pollyanna childhood and such a warm and loving family sound to the world?" Too perfect? Probably. Definitely. As slightly unreal as it does sound, the truth is that it was and is pretty ideal. Human, with ups and downs, some days better than others, but, overall, hard to beat for security and learning, love and good times. How did that happen? I think we were basically brought up on "the power of positive thinking" model. Mother and Daddy had high expectations for us and were strict, but always reinforced that they loved us no matter how well or poorly we did. They believed strongly in our good character and our ability to succeed at something we were willing to focus on and work hard for. The disciplinary model was that we might do a bad thing, but we were never a bad person. If we were rude or transgressed in some way, we usually were sent to our room where one of our parents would come to ask, disappointedly, why we would do such a thing when we were such a fine and good person. Once "the talk" was over, we were immediately accepted back into whatever was going on in the house and the subject was never spoken of again. There were no grudges, just an effort for clear and swift resolution. There was a very strong sense that we were all part of this indissoluble caring family together and that everything we did not only reflected on us, but on the whole. Fighting was not tolerated. The message was that we should be smart enough to work things out by talking them through. I don't recall conflict in the house. Mother and Daddy are bound to have had strong differences of opinion along sixty-plus years of marriage, but I never once heard them yell or argue angrily. They showed unwavering respect for each other and for us. We were never demeaned or made to feel foolish in any way. Mother used to say that if you back someone into a corner, he has no choice but to fight. We were not backed into corners. One key element, I believe, to our future self-confidence was our parents' acceptance that each of us had different strengths. Their encouragement was to be the best we could be; but every effort was made not to compare us to each other. We naturally did enough of that on our own. During my early school years, I was never shown my national or comparative achievement test scores. I believe that is because they were quite low compared to my siblings and they wanted to allow for the fact that I might be a late bloomer. They did not show me the depressing results and thus allowed me to believe in myself until I finally caught on and bloomed after all. A wise person said, "Children do what you do, not what you say." Growing up in this home over the years has put us in the habit of getting along in these same ways now. Our upbringing has everything to do with the positive way we are trying to deal with Mother and each other during this tough time. It is almost scary to realize how deeply influenced and formed we have been from our years of living with them and how amazingly lucky we were that the influence was a positive one.

4
THIRD TRIP BACK HOME

The circle. Wow! How it seems to roll on. Today was amazing! We are gathering again. Coming together as a family. Homing back in on this house from wherever we are. I could feel the energy building—and sure enough, it was a totally momentous occasion. Daddy didn't call it Headlong Hall for nothing. I think the best fruit of our gathering this time was the expansive sense of celebration, of tremendous relief and very real joy that this mother we all love has had a pretty perfect move thus far. It has all gone better than our wildest dreams and she has been such a trooper—making friends, interacting, rising to the potential. Those are her "quarters" now. Change partners and dance. Life goes on.

For the rest of us, life is going on too. As we look toward dissolving family gatherings in this house, it was only fitting that we come together here again. We have all had countless family dinners here. Celebrated holidays. Celebrated big life moments. Now we celebrate the Jane and Jimmy Hughes years— who they were, what they stood for, how we loved them, and what they gave to each of us large and small.

What could be more perfect than a big family Sunday midday luncheon—which was a weekly prerequisite, lo, these many years. The best fun was the fact that as we have sorted and delved into all the far corners of this house, period pieces have surfaced which have caught the imagination of the sorters.

Before we knew it, we were thinking these must be a part of the gathering—and what a gathering it was!

The family that was in town began to gather about eleven-thirty. From then on, this house was caught up in a froth of activity—a state it had enjoyed many times through the years. Each time the door opened, the new arrival would enter amid hugs and greetings and then get into the spirit of the thing. It wouldn't be long before he or she would turn up in some form of costume. Anne and Elizabeth had come to town. Anne turned out in swags of pink tulle with accompanying large black velvet hat while Elizabeth donned a Mexican embroidered sundress with appliquéd sweater—quite chic. Anne Sayle appeared in a purple ruffled Spanish *senorita* number that one of us had worn at Hutchison School May Day. She was searching for ways to close the placket. No problem, we used Mother's hearing aid wire piece to span the gap quite nicely. She had responded to the call of the odd earrings and was sporting five very different and intriguing ones. They showed off nicely against her black hair. Jane was a study in cross cultures, appearing in an only slightly ripped, embroidered kimono, but unable to resist adding a fur neck piece and a very pink pillbox hat made entirely of large rose blossoms. Janie Sayle had on an extravagant white '50s semiformal with full net skirt and red velvet trimmings. Little Mary Catherine and Caroline had so much fun choosing that every time you would see them they were in an exotic new get-up. Catherine immediately dove into the scene and emerged in a long pink satin skirt and exotic velvet evening cape. I had fallen out laughing over an old cocktail dress I'd found in Mother's sewing closet which looked fine from the front, but which had the skirt ripped totally off in the back.

Only the zipper hung down from the waist. I couldn't resist wearing it and did so over my running tights. The look was greatly enhanced by the mink collar I wore. A tiny red hat with red netting covered my face. I held one of Daddy's pipes in my teeth, and wore huge crystal chandelier earrings that hurt like hell. The boys got on the bandwagon by lunchtime (although I admit it took them a while to see if this dress up thing was for real). The spirit of the thing just took on a life of its own. Jim ended up in two top hats wielding a very large club he had found in the attic guaranteed to fell a man with a single blow. Allen Jr. wore a hat that he had jerryrigged to look as though an arrow had gone through his head! Robert donned on old white summer tux and Dick put on a shiny green top hat for his outfit. It was the least he could do when baby Will and even 6-week-old Allen III had on hats! They also chewed on a couple of Daddy's pipes! Laurie arrived a bit after the rest. You had to love her natural response to the scene of, "I've got to find an outfit!" She did, too, and made us all jealous when she put on Mother's old satin evening gown—all on the bias, natch, and actually got it zipped—and she the mother of a newborn to boot!

We asked Mother's helper to come outside and take one large group tableau on the front lawn with the house as backdrop. It sure looked to me as though the camera was held at a crazy angle, but maybe that will just add to the scene. We all laughed when the joggers and walkers passed by, but probably not as hard as they were laughing when they saw us. Someone was heard to say, "This family can even make cleaning out the attic fun!" Someone else was heard to ask in a whisper if Mother had passed away!

As you might imagine, we were all in high spirits and lunch was so much fun. We all squeezed around the table—so full of laughter and interaction as it has always been—just as it should be. I smiled. All of us there because of Mother and Daddy. Connected. The circle.

Little six-year-old Caroline said grace as we all held hands. That little husky voice of hers saying grace brought the tears to my eyes. It seemed so right to have this fresh young one, full of all the potential that Mother and Daddy could pass on to her, carrying their torch along now that they can no more. Wonderful immortality.

We asked the question, "What do you remember most here?" and took turns, young and old, around the table answering it one by one as the others listened. Mother playing Mah Jong with Catherine, especially on snowy days. Peanut butter and pickle sandwiches. "First Dibs!" and stampeding to the piano to practice after dinner. Bernice passing the platters of rice and vegetables every night and rolling her eyes if we winked at her. Sitting on top of the warm dishwasher listening to "The Shadow" with her on the kitchen radio after supper. How much we each loved her, young and old. Playing with the buzzer under the table that rang out in the kitchen when we needed something. The silver tray from which Daddy "served" our mandatory shots to go to camp each June. Daddy backing into cars on the turnaround. Naming our rabbit Rabbit E. Lee. Sunday ravioli suppers. Mother telling how she was asked to train to run the hurtles for America in the Olympics and her parents flatly refusing to allow her to do such an outrageous thing. Mother lost in her world of raking leaves. Allen, Jr. as a child being allowed to play the mad scientist at the kitchen sink with Mother's food coloring set and countless little bottles. Our parrot Lorito laughing raucously and loudly calling for Mother from his kitchen perch. Daddy giving my yearly October 12th birthday toast—"Here's to the day Columbus discovered the world, and the world discovered Sally!" The boyhood stories Daddy told of **canoeing** the great Mississippi River from Memphis to New Orleans with his brothers. Lively storytelling always around this dinner table. Laughing. Never being able to wear hair rollers or tee shirts to the table. Children slipping underneath the table after dessert and thinking they were hiding, grabbing the big folks feet to loud exclamations. Donovan leaning back once again in the antique chair and breaking it, followed by Mother blessing me out for not bringing him up better. Begging Allen to rough-house with us after supper and Mother calling after us that someone was going to end up crying. Daddy pushing back his chair after dinner when I was little and patting his legs for me to come sit on his lap. Dick wowing ever brilliant Daddy by supplying some obscure date Daddy could not recall and never telling Daddy that he'd just happened to hear it on Jeopardy the night before! The whole day was saturated in memories that each of us has had in this great "heart home." We were all aware of the fullness of it. A close family enjoying each other and doing our best to navigate through this upheaval and change with warmth and appreciation.

One theme I noticed in the comments was our parents' undivided attention to each of us. Mother always said that that was what a child really craves—your undivided attention and she managed to give us a lot of it.

We also took turns telling, or rather confessing, what was the

WORST thing we ever did in this house. It was pretty revealing and hysterical but I just can't keep my eyes open anymore to tell you all of it. I will say that Elizabeth brought the house down when she gave her one-word answer, "Slouch."

❦❦❦ ❦❦❦ ❦❦❦ ❦❦❦

What an amazing night! But which night? They are all crowding in on one another so fast. Everything in a hurry piling in on each other—so much to do. You can see it in the handwriting. Just look. We are so busy with the house, but the real news is Mother.

Mother—all calm. All perfectly happy rearranging her dresser. Wanting to introduce us to her new friends. How lucky can we be? The truth of that sinks down slowly into my being. It is seriously wonderful that she is responding like this. It could have been World War III or a meltdown. Seeing her get so much more interaction is wonderful. Today was a great example. Jane and I were walking Mother on one of the garden paths when out into the garden came Dan, a dapper gentleman who must have done wartime work for the CIA. He is always planning secret meetings and asking, with a piercing look, if you are coming. He was dressed for an outing complete with hat and overcoat. When Mother saw him coming she stopped and said brightly, "Oh, here is my friend!" They clasped hands and kissed cheeks like long lost friends. He then announced, "I'm off to walk down Front Street. I think I may run into my mother." We called out to please tell her "Hello" for us and he was very appreciative. I was enchanted and told Jane on the side that that particular garden path would henceforth and forever be "Front Street" to me. Not five minutes later, we ran into Dan again inside and what do you suppose? The whole cheery interaction was repeated with hugs and hand clasping. However, instead of visiting his mother, he was intensely planning a "very important meeting." Then he was off again. Think of how nice to be welcomed enthusiastically and warmly this way, on and off, all day long—each time fresh and new. Mother may not do names anymore, but she speaks to everyone, clearly enjoys people, and they sense it. The habit of good manners has stood her in good stead.

Each night we go out and put her to bed. It is a great time of the day. The hustle and bustle of sorting and organizing the house, getting down and dirty, is behind us. We have taken that most welcome and needed thing—a bath! We head out to her at dusk, all refreshed. The drive out creates that still moment when the magnitude of what is happening sinks in. Not only that our journey with Mother has come so far, but also just the sheer volume of how much progress we are making organizing Headlong Hall. It is laborious but it is getting done—and so much faster than any of us thought it could be.

Mother is so happy to see us. She just lights up. We visit a bit before we help her into her nightgown, reaching down inside the sleeves to take her hand and guide it through, just like a baby's. Jane reads *Dorcus Porcus* tonight and we all laugh when the little pig Dorcus Porcus gets loose in the ladies' sewing bee and hides under the minister's wife's skirts. Mother loved it. We are still reaching Mother with the simple nursery rhymes of her childhood. Then, with the lights out, we sing the soft, low lullabies she taught us and snuggle with her. It is a very peaceful time and there is no question that it comforts us every bit as much as it does her.

The Studio has been looming over us ever since we have known that one day we would have to sort through and reclaim it. It is a large, den-like room looking out onto the back lawn. It has fireplace and kitchenette, dressing room and bath. It was added on when Grandmother stopped coming over to our house each morning and going to her own home after supper and completely moved in hook, line and sinker. Her big old bed was there, the desk, lots of books. She died peacefully in that room with her old caretaker Seebelle quietly quilting beside the bed. At the last, Seebelle was working on a quilt she called "A Mean Row to Hoe" and I guess that's how she felt about things just then.

Since then, Mother stopped calling it "Wa-Wa's Emporium" and has called the room "The Studio" as she envisioned doing her painting there. Along the way, it has served in various other capacities from "Honeymoon Haven" (for newly-wed children come to visit) to "The Casbah" (for Donovan's summer bachelor digs). It has gathered items for each of these roles as the years have passed. Now it is a cleanup job of awesome proportions. The large closets built into the paneling are now full of all sorts of things. They range from the boxes of pottery Mother had brought home from Mexico in the '50s and never unpacked, to a plethora of framed diplomas spanning one-hundred-and-fifty years. Anne's painting area of recent years holds down one large corner. All of this we are brave enough to launch into . . . or are we?

Allen tunes the radio to the "oldies but goodies" station. We get on our grubbies and we start in bit by bit. This is all very healthy stuff we are doing. Now that I think of it, a shrink would definitely approve. By handling and processing each and every piece of this horde of family things over days and days we are also dealing with it emotionally. Comments pop out amid the general activity. "Oh, do you remember this?" or "What a riot! I don't think I've ever seen this silly thing." or "Please! Do you want to join me in a ceremonial ditching of this yucky thing? I have wanted to chunk it for years." or "Look at this. It is a real treasure." or "Don't throw that away! I always loved it. Anne and I used to make weird hairdos with it when we were little." "Look at this old photograph. This man looks a lot like Taylor." So it goes as we slowly say good-bye. I've handled so many old books passed down through the ages (Wow! Did my family love to read!). It makes me want to write in every book I ever give from now on. I find I'm very disappointed when I open a particularly fat lovely one and find no inscription. "Charles Gordon Frierson, 1870," "Jimmy, with love from Aunt Pearl," "To Edna from your dear friend Kate Chopin, Christmas, Saint Louis," "Nathaniel from Mother, Windy Crest, Michigan"—I feel I'm getting to know these ancestors a bit. Part of a chain of command that has now passed down to me. I must do as well as I can with it, and then in turn pass it on again.

Just the time spent in the trenches with each other is therapeutic. Just the steady stream of one item after another looked at, decided on, kept to choose later, or tossed out to go start a new life somewhere else. Looking at each thing not through the eyes of whether we want it or not, but rather is there any of the four of us that might want it? That shows how far we've come, looking with eyes that want each person to have anything that would give him or her pleasure whether we think it is an item worth keeping or not. After all, who am I to say?

We are getting the job done, but the key is we are sharing the experience and having fun with it. What a waste if we did not! When will we be together quite like this ever again? Steeped in our childhood memories with the very people we lived them with. We are closing the chapter we began together. The circle. The strong, ever changing, ever growing circle. Us.

⊄⊃ ⊄⊃ ⊄⊃ ⊄⊃

There is much more ahead of us, dividing up this house and its treasures, making group decisions. How we'll do, I do not know. I have heard it said that in sharing an inheritance or a lifeboat you sometimes learn more than you want to know about another person. My dearest hope is that we will somehow be secure enough to take the higher ground. That we will be smart enough to remember that long after these possessions are divvied up, we will still be brother and sisters. Relationships that have the power to carry and sustain us through our whole lifetimes are what is at risk here. Even the closest of families have derailed during this kind of stressful time when everyone is tired, overwhelmed, and emotions run high. I do know that our parents would and should be ashamed of us if we stoop to falling out over mere possessions. It scares me a little. The next few months will tell and I will be glad when they are behind us.

5
PASSING THE BATON
BACK TO CHARLESTON

My own home. I round the corner after my fourteen-hour drive from Mother's and there is my house waiting for me. How good it feels to be home. Unloading, I carry an arm load of wonderful old hats that Mother and Daddy used to wear into the house. For whatever reason, this triggers a sudden clutch inside me and wracking sobs. I am distraught. I feel the reality of their things, their memories—their very identity being dispersed, absorbed into each of us, even fading away! Some going to this house, some to others. Like they are being erased. I can hardly stand the thought. The wellspring is empty. There is no longer that font to return to from any time or place; to always be welcomed, fed, listened to, recharged. Now WE are the wellspring. We are what is left. We have to feed ourselves. We and our own children are part of the new wellspring. My tears come hard. Very hard.

Somehow when we were choosing and packing in the big house it all seemed okay. The things were in their own setting. Now Daddy's general's hat looks at me from the pile of luggage in my hall and Mother's navy straw Easter bonnet can't hold its own in the bright sunlight coming through my window. The tiny white blossoms seeming tired and dingy.

Maybe this is osmosis. Maybe these sobs are the beginning

of my realizing that we are taking in all that they were and somehow incorporating it into what and who we are. We are us and our parents and all who came before, back to The Garden of Eden. It is our turn and it is a big responsibility. We are all grown up. I feel as though someone has thrust a baton into my outstretched hand and sent me the message that it is my brief time to carry the torch, that life is fleeting. Give it all you've got, we've given you all we can in blood and brains to run a good race—now go for it with all you've got and then be willing to pass the baton to the next person for their turn. The tears slowly stop. This is life. I know these things, have known these things, even though I have never felt the piercing reality of them ever before quite as I do now carrying in an arm load of old hats. This is what we are all born to do and no one could ask for parents who taught the way better through word and deed. I might be ready. I even have time. Look what Keats did in a few short years—or Van Gogh—or whoever wanted something enough to make it happen. I want to take all that I am and pour it out in living and painting and loving until I am all used up. I am so grateful that they have given me the tools. Until I, too, must pass the baton—and on—and on. Another link in a long chain. A circle. The circle.

6
CLOSING

I cannot write in this journal again. I am all dried up. I somehow sense that my feelings and thoughts have run their course through this passage. And what a passage it has been! What a lesson in growing up, slowing down to listen, adapting, trying to make it work for everyone, though sometimes failing. Feeling good, feeling sad; having fun with people you love, getting overtired; seeing things through other people's eyes; acting generous, acting petty; feeling acutely aware of life passing swiftly, yet aware too of all there is left to live. Trying to keep the big picture in mind, making lemonade out of lemons—doing our best to carry on the legacy of our amazing parents. I feel like the salmon, swimming upstream, who gathers all she has in her and pours it out to accomplish an important and overwhelming task, then falls back totally spent. I feel like that. I want a field to lie fallow in. I want to be home in the here and now and sink into the arms of the beautiful life I have been blessed with. I want to canter a horse through the wintry woods and spend days lost in my painting. I want to be with my children. I know that I am more after this journey. How much more or how different, I can't tell yet. My focus on all of these changes has been so powerful and absorbing that I find I need to get to know myself a little better again, now that life can settle down. I need to get comfortable in my new skin. I need to be still and ask myself what I want to do with my one precious life. I want to float free for a while and see what rises to the top. What do they say? "You have to lose it to find it." I started my journey upset and worried about this passage and all the sadness that it would mean. I have ended up finding and gaining so much—with a much deeper appreciation for Mother, Headlong Hall, my family, and what is at stake. It was not lost. In a sense it is more "found" than it ever was before. We did not unravel the tapestry of our old family home and life, we made it stronger, more realistic, and more full of life. Rebirth. The circle. Thank you, Daddy. Thank you, Mother.

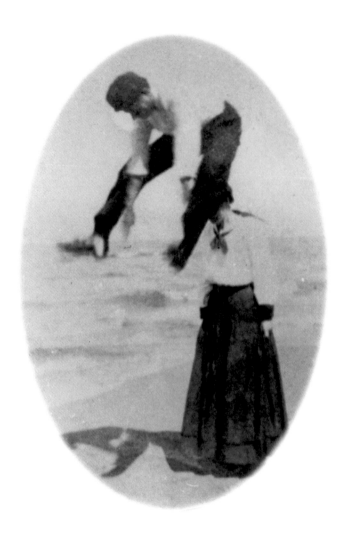

SOME OF WHAT I LEARNED THAT MAY HELP OTHERS ON THEIR JOURNEY
Overview and Practicalities

Overview:

It is with humility that I undertake offering suggestions. I am not trained in this field. I do not even know exactly why these things worked well for us, I am only deeply thankful that they did. This was my personal journey and not all situations are the same; still, some threads of truth will strike home. My purpose is to be of some use to you in your rite of passage with your parents or in preparing your children for your own transition. I do believe that there were certain fundamentals that helped position us for success and as such, I will try to pass them on.

* There are many things I learned along the way, but I must start by saying that by far the most important thing was the spirit in which this overwhelming task was taken on. It is a difficult time by any standards and it is much easier if one realizes that relationships are the most important thing. Concentrate on being open-minded to the other siblings helping you make decisions. Treat them with respect and care. Long after the parent is gone, you and your siblings are left in this world together and this is the real legacy that is left to you. Beware that the stresses of decision

making do not undermine the relationships that can have the power to sustain you in the years to come. Filter your actions and comments through this awareness.

* You may have heard these words before, but they are really worth hearing again as this difficult time unfolds. Happiness is a choice we make. No one is responsible for our own happiness but ourselves. Don't let these events bring you down.

* Be easy on yourself. Try to keep balance in your life and not let the new situation overwhelm you. Realize that it is going to to be a long endeavor and take it one baby step at a time. Keeping a journal during this time helped me to keep my perspective.

* Take care of yourself. Good health and attitude is key to any successful undertaking.

* Pace yourself or you will get burnt out. Save time for friends and hobbies.

* Remember the power of laughter and indulge yourself to the fullest!

* Remember that there is no "only" way to a solution. There is no absolute right or wrong.

* It is hard, but try to stay flexible. The playing field is always changing in this task. In our caretaking of C.D.'s mother, I recall thinking we had solved a great problem and relaxed in satisfaction, only to find a few days later that it was no longer working. We needed to adapt and come up with a new solution, which would also become obsolete sooner

rather than later. This pattern repeated itself many times. It can be frustrating.

* In problem solving, realize that the one thing you cannot do is fix everything and make it right again. You cannot make that person young again. You cannot bring back their clear thinking. What you CAN do is give them their best chance of enjoying the life they have left.

* Get rid of guilt. One of the real ironies of caregiving is that you never feel that you have given enough. No matter how much one gives, there is always more that could be done. This is hard, but this is where you need to be realistic. One thing that helps is to think of what you are doing in your own life and ask yourself how much your parent, if they were in their best state of mind, would really want you to give it up to care for them. Usually the answer will give you some peace.

* Appreciate that they can still give a lot even through the fog . . . the hand held, the odd comment that does make sense. My mother taught me a lot about living in the days she was turning back into a child.

* A huge gift to you and me through all of this is AWARENESS. This is so major. Watching a parent unravel is a reminder of our own mortality and our own potential in this life. Open yourself to this powerful awareness to be more alive to go after your dreams, mend relationships, and to live more fully every day in the time you have left.

* As tough as it is to deal with an aging parent, talking to friends who lost their parent when they were young brings

home the reality of how truly lucky we are to have our current problem, after a lifetime of having our parents, and not the one of early loss that they have had to live with for so long.

* Woody Allen once said, "I don't mind dying. I just don't want to be there when it happens." In some ways, dementia and senility are a protection against the indignities that old age can bring. The parent is not really there when they happen. I wish my wonderful mother were as bright and sharp as she always was, but if she can't be, this thought that she is protected in some way from her bitter realities comforts me.

* Whatever your beliefs, a spiritual life can give one strength and peace as nothing else can.

Practicalities:

* Look at your parent's and family's situation and begin to get an overview of what is needed to care for your parent and how this fits into the family picture. Think what the parent can still respond to and enjoy and what concrete medical support is needed. The earlier you start, the more feeling of self-control you will have.

* Begin to fact-find with no preconceived prejudices. Look at all the options, call homes for the elderly and other facilities to see if they offer the level of care that is needed and can be afforded. Make an appointment and get a feel for a place, atmosphere, and the people there. Listen to

your instincts. If time is not a factor, volunteering in a place can give one a close-up view of what really goes on and if residents are happy there.

* Meet with the decision making part of the family and put all the options out there for discussion. Listen to every-one's opinion even if you disagree. We began these talks by saying how thankful we were for this great family and for each other. This helped us focus on the big picture and being sure everyone was on board with the plans as they unfolded.

* Delegate and organize. Any plan can be broken down into smaller tasks that can be divided up among the responsible decision makers. This not only spreads the work load, but people also buy into something more if they are a part of making it happen and realize what goes into making it happen.

* One of the most critical tasks is to begin to gather impor-tant papers. The parent will never remember more than they do now, so try and find out as much as you can before they can no longer recall where things are. Locate and make copies of, among other things: birth certificate, safe-ty deposit box location and key, marriage license, military discharge papers, deeds to property and other official pa-pers, bank accounts, medical records, social security card, valuables, names and numbers of important contacts such as lawyer, minister, insurance agent, retirement fund con-tact, etc. The MOST important papers, **after an updated and valid will**, are advance directives and a durable power of attorney and a copy of these should be in the hands

of you, the lawyer, and any caregiver at all times. Advance directives (living will and durable power of attorney for health care) can state your parent's end of life wishes and provide legal protection from such things as being resuscitated when they are basically in a vegetable state. A durable power of attorney gives a designated person the right to make other legally binding decisions for a parent should they become incapacitated. Getting down the identities of who people were in our old family photographs was something we only partly did. Now there is no one else to ask. I cannot suggest strongly enough that you consider getting this same information organized on yourself and giving it to your own children while you are able.

* We continually tried to make decisions based on what we thought our mother would like best. The irony here is that in her new state of confusion many things that would have mattered to her were no longer on her screen. Once we realized this it was easier to be relaxed.

* Keeping a parent at home, whether it is in yours or in theirs, is really more isolating than one would think at first glance. It usually means attendants and not the level of social interaction on a regular basis that a really good assisted living home can offer. The perception in our age group is that it is always nicer to keep a parent at home if one can. My belief is that, though it sounds good, in practice this is often not the best decision.

* We found that the timing of Mother's move was all important. She was alert enough to enjoy social interaction and benefit from outings, but too fuzzy to reject the move

out of her home. We wondered if she knew it on some subconscious level, but it did not affect the move.

* Mother used to say that we have only so much room in our brains and it is up to us to fill it with good things or bad. Acting on this premise, we surrounded Mother with happy things . . . Disney movies she could still relate to because the stories were age old, uplifting music, old movies. Regular TV and radio with their drama and conflict were off limits.

* Enjoy your confused parent however you can. We could still connect with Mother for a long time through touch, the old songs she had sung us so often, and nursery rhymes from her childhood. Take whatever you can and enjoy the contact because in our case it was not long before that connection too was gone.

* A plan that worked well for us was to spend a lot of time at the new assisted living place before Mother moved in so that she felt very much at home and comfortable there. She would spend the morning there on and off for several days, then the whole day, then stay for dinner. By the time she moved in, she was used to it and happy with being there.

* Having the new assisted living home room look as much like Mother's at home with familiar things in it, I believe, made her transition much more comfortable mentally, emotionally, and physically.

* Be glad if your parent has developed the "habit" of good manners and a basically happy personality. Even when

my Mother was so confused that she could hardly say my name, her pleasant demeanor made her friends of her caretakers in the home and her contemporaries there. Her main caregiver ended up calling her "Mama" and it meant a lot to know that she was giving her steady affection even when we were not there to give it.

* Personalities can change in older people as happened to C.D.'s mother. She would say angry things to me from time to time. Once I realized that she was not her real self and that she knew she could strike out at me in her frustration because I was "safe" and would never leave her, I could let it go.

* Diversion became a powerful and happy way to deal with my confused parent. We avoided confrontation. There was nothing to be gained from it since she was no longer able to understand an explanation. Put "diversion" in your toolbox and use it often.

* Sorting and handling all the family possessions with your family is a highly therapeutic process. Here you have a chance to say goodbye to the life you lived in that home and do it with the people you grew up with. When it got to dividing up things, we discussed and set up simple ground rules in advance. We had a clear and early understanding of the system before we put it into action. No one talked about what they hoped to get or made anyone feel pressured not to pick an item they wanted. We got back any item that we had given them or that had our name in it. We decided what went in sets, and what was separate, ahead of time. We did not have any appraisals, we chose on affec-

tion for the item, not monetary value. This has turned out to be a very good decision as many times an item of small value has been chosen long before one of great value for sentimental reasons. On her second pick among lovely old silver pieces to pick from, Anne chose a small silver piece that used to sit on the coffee table and that she had loved to play with as a child. It meant more to her than all the more flamboyant pieces. I'm glad that we chose rather than have things left outright to us, because I have ended up with the things that mean the most to me personally and my siblings have too. We took turns 1-2-3-4-4-3-2-1, up and down the scale, until no one wanted anything anymore. Allen suggested that we put four numbers on paper bits and put them in a bowl; then he held the bowl high in the air and had each sibling pick one, and we began in that order. Fair. Fair. Fair.

Here is an excerpt from my journal pages that shows how it worked for us:

Monday was 'choose the linens' day. Jane and I got up early and tried to remember just where we'd put them all, but not before we had that blessed first cup of coffee. Lots of trips up and down the stairs produced linens of every type and description covering all the open spaces and furniture of the living room. Bed linens on the baby grand piano, tablecloths and their napkins on the love seats, toppers on the fire screens, runners on the Mah Jong table, handtowels on the sofa, embroidered napkins on the coffee table. Odd bread covers with delicious lace edging and pale blue embroidery on the end table, placemats and casual tablecloths under the French windows. It was a real scene. Something of every type of fine handwork here. It spoke volumes of the Phillips ladies' love of fine handwork, both their own and others.

Marily picked the linens for Allen since he is not exactly into them and it was fun. We were all loaded up with linens an hour or so later when Marily looked around and said that she couldn't see another thing she wanted to pick and was through. But the real fun started when she came back into the room a bit later and some embroidered napkins caught her eye and she thought maybe she'd just have one more pick and then quit. It was something we could all relate to. She was laughing and so were we. A few turns later a couple of monogrammed handtowels began to look good to her and back in she came for those. We were all enjoying each other. It does take on a life of it's own and the comments toward the end were wonderful. 'I must be through!' 'Well, I think Ellen just might like that organdy baby pillowcase.' 'This is so pretty. Would these stains ever come out?' 'Who is going to iron all this stuff?' 'I guess Annie really might be able to use that tablecloth. I hear that style is coming back.' 'Do any of your children have double beds?' 'I guess you could make a pretty lingerie case out of that table runner.' 'This is gorgeous, but what would you use it for?' The answers were pretty rare. We knew it was time to stop when we started choosing lace edged linen hand towels to use as doll bed sheets for grandaughters we didn't even have yet!

* Finding some closure after moving everything out of our old house was a problem for me. Most of the things went to my children, which made us all happy, but I had some of Mother's clothes that I just couldn't seem to part with quite yet. A great solution came for me in the idea to have a party to celebrate my mother and then I would pass on the things to a costume department. I planned a ladies tea party where I live in Charleston. I used Mother's tiny engraved note cards as invitations and wrote, "You are your mother and moving mine out of our family home has proven it

to me. Come dressed as your mother and let's celebrate them and us!" When the day came, C.D. had copied a lovely photo of Mother's face and put it on every photograph in the whole house. One chandelier was covered in old long white gloves while the other was covered in 1920's hats and thick-soled shoes. Dresses from different stages in Mother's life hung along the dining room wall. The bartender came to me exasperated with the news that there was plenty of everything on the bar to make any sort of drink, but only teacups to serve it in! I said, "That's right. Our guests can have whatever they want to drink today, but only out of teacups." The table was laid as for a high tea, but white and red wine filled the tea and coffee pots. I dressed in one of Mother's dresses and hats from the 1940's and greeted my guests as they came in . . . and what a procession they made! I marveled at their outfits and how enthusiastically they embrased the spirit of the party. One had died her hair totally white for the occasion and was going to meet her husband later for dinner and surprise him, another wore a sign that said " My name is Sue. Please return me to room 24." Another came in a 1950's bathing suit carrying a crab net with zinc oxide smeared on her nose, while another usually conservative friend came as her flambouyant mother in slinkly black dress, long flowing hair that we had never seen down before, and carrying a dramatically long cigarette holder! There were many marvelous outfits. It was a priceless afternoon of bonding, laughing, getting teary-eyed, and talking about our mothers in a highly therapeutic way. Once it was over, I could let those clothes move on. Anne has dealt with her closure by using material from Mother's sewing room to make hundreds of tiny angel dolls and taking them to people all over the world when she goes on mission trips.

* Reading selected chapters of *How To Care For Aging Parents* by Virginia Morris gave very sensible and specific information on caring for aging parents and the issues surrounding this challenge. I recommend the book highly.

* I would invite your additions to this list of suggestions. There may be suggestions that you have discovered in your different situations that would help others to know. Please feel free to e-mail suggestions to *thecircle@musc.edu*. In our next printing we may be able to touch more people with your helpful ideas.

Good luck on the journey and may the circle be unbroken!

ABOUT THE AUTHOR

Sally Hughes Smith is a painter and a published author and illustrator. She grew up in Memphis, Tennessee and graduated from Duke University with a major in English. She now lives in Charleston, South Carolina where she and her husband, a pediatric surgeon, have reared their four children.

www.sallysmith.com